SpringerBriefs in Applied Sciences and Technology

Nanotheranostics

Series editors

Subramanian Tamil Selvan, Singapore, Singapore
Karthikeyan Narayanan, Singapore, Singapore
Padmanabhan Parasuraman, Singapore, Singapore
Paulmurugan Ramasamy, Palo Alto, USA

More information about this series at http://www.springer.com/series/13040

Atefeh Zarepour · Ali Zarrabi
Arezoo Khosravi

SPIONs as
Nano-Theranostics Agents

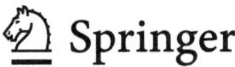 Springer

Atefeh Zarepour
Department of Biotechnology, Faculty of
 Advanced Sciences and Technologies
University of Isfahan
Isfahan
Iran

Arezoo Khosravi
Department of Mechanical Engineering,
 Khomeinishahr Branch
Islamic Azad University
Khomeinishahr, Isfahan
Iran

Ali Zarrabi
Department of Biotechnology, Faculty of
 Advanced Sciences and Technologies
University of Isfahan
Isfahan
Iran

ISSN 2191-530X   ISSN 2191-5318   (electronic)
SpringerBriefs in Applied Sciences and Technology
ISSN 2197-6740   ISSN 2197-6759   (electronic)
Nanotheranostics
ISBN 978-981-10-3562-3   ISBN 978-981-10-3563-0   (eBook)
DOI 10.1007/978-981-10-3563-0

Library of Congress Control Number: 2016961676

Printed on acid-free paper

This Springer imprint is published by Springer Nature
The registered company is Springer Nature Singapore Pte Ltd.
The registered company address is: 152 Beach Road, #22-06/08 Gateway East, Singapore 189721, Singapore

Contents

Abbreviations

AMF	Alternating magnetic field
CTCs	Circulating tumor cells
EPR	Enhanced permeability and retention
FA	Folic acid
FGF	Fibroblast growth factor
FITC	Fluorescein isothiocyanate
GO	Graphene oxide
HPG	Hyperbranched polyglycerol
HSA	Human serum albumin
MCLs	Magnetic cationic liposomes
MNPs	Magnetic nanoparticles
MRI	Magnetic resonance imaging
MS	Multiple sclerosis
NIR	Near-infrared
NMR	Nuclear magnetic resonance
PA	Photoacoustic
PDT	Photodynamic therapy
PEG	Polyethylene glycol
PEI	Polyethylenimine
PGA	Polyglycolic acid
PLA	Polylactic acid
PLGA	Polylactic glycolic acid
PNIPAAM	Poly(N-isopropylacrylamide)
PTA	Photothermal absorber
PTT	Photothermal therapy
PVA	Polyvinyl alcohol
PVCL	Poly(N-vinylcaprolactam)
rGO	Reduced graphene oxide
ROS	Reactive oxygen species
SDT	Sonodynamic therapy

SERS   Surface-enhanced Raman spectroscopy
siRNA   Small interfering ribonucleic acid
SPIONs   Superparamagnetic iron oxide nanoparticles

List of Figures

Chapter 1
SPIONs as Nano-Theranostics Agents

1.1 Introduction

Nowadays, cancer is known as one of the most causes of human death in the world and so many efforts have been conducted to identify a useful method of treatment. Cancer is a heterogeneous and adaptable disease, which makes it essential to study diverse types of treatments depending on patient characteristics and disease progression. Over the years, scientists have developed various methods of cancer treatment including surgery, chemotherapy, and radiotherapy. Despite the many attempts that have been made in this area, there is still no considerable success in the treatment of cancer and it usually fails because of cancer recurrence and metastasis [1–4]. Surgery, as the most important approach for removing solid tumors is very invasive and has limitations such as unpleasant condition for patients and hardly elimination of all tumor cells especially in the metastatic case. On the other hand, chemotherapy and radiotherapy have not been successful due to their limited therapeutic effects, serious side effects on normal cells and adjacent tissues, and the risk of drug resistance. Thus, development of novel strategy for cancer treatment with less side effect, lower cost, and optimal therapeutic efficacy is demanding [5–9].

Except cancer, other inflammatory diseases, like neurodegenerative disease, diabetes, and atherosclerosis also need an effective therapeutic approach which provides the highest efficiency and the lowest side effect of drugs.

Nanotechnology is one of the novel technologies which has the potential to be used in the treatment of different diseases. Nanotechnology has become one of the critical research endeavors of the twenty-first century and its widespread application in various fields and disciplines, specifically in health care which is named as nanomedicine, is becoming increasingly applicable which may even replace the conventional medicines [1, 10–12].

Nanomaterials are materials with at least one dimension in the size of nanometer (10^{-9} m). The materials' size reduction from bulk to nano range causes an alteration

© The Author(s) 2017
A. Zarepour et al., *SPIONs as Nano-Theranostics Agents*,
Nanotheranostics, DOI 10.1007/978-981-10-3563-0_1

in their properties or introduction of new properties which makes them good candidates for medical applications. For example, their nanometric size prevents them from kidneys clearance and therefore extends their circulation in the blood pool depending on their surface functional characteristics. Moreover, they have high reactive surface for loading of drugs/imaging agents/targeting agents [13–18].

Nanoparticles are materials with three dimensions in the nano range (1–100 nm) and a highly active surface in comparison to other nanomaterials which has been extensively studied in the field of nanomedicine. They can act as carriers for drugs in drug delivery systems, as well as being a self-medication in some cases. They can easily travel all over the body through the bloodstream without being recognized by the immune system, transmit through the vessels, penetrate to the tissues, and deliver their cargo to the targeted cells [19–23].

The surface of these particles could be engineered with different polymers that not only improve their biocompatibility, but also increase their drug loading ability and provide a broad area for attachment of different imaging and targeting agents. Binding targeting factors reduces the drug side effects and increases the drug's effectiveness by delivering them to the targeted tissues. The inclusion of imaging and therapeutic agents together within a nanosystem introduces a new field in medicine named theranostic nanomedicine [24–28].

John Funkhouser coined the term of theranostic in 2002 in one of his reviews. Theranostics combine therapeutic and diagnostic features into one optimal platform that could overcome the undesirable differences in biodistribution and selectivity that exist between distinct imaging and therapeutic agents. It has potential application in personalized medicine which results to tailor a treatment regimen producing improved outcomes, reduced costs, and fewer side effects. Moreover, it could monitor and evaluate the therapeutic efficacy during the treatment period which accelerates therapeutic decisions [29, 30].

Among various types of nanoparticles, magnetic nanoparticles[1] with the desired imaging sensitivity and therapeutic efficacy could be the most promising probes for theranostics and more specifically in nano-theranostics. Iron oxide nanoparticles, magnetite (Fe_3O_4) and maghemit (γ-Fe_2O_3), because of their unique properties such as biocompatibility and biodegradability are the most attractive type of MNPs that could be applied in nano-theranostics applications. They are employed in numerous biomedical applications such as magnetic separation, drug and gene delivery, cancer hyperthermia, and magnetic resonance imaging (MRI).[2] Fe_3O_4 nanoparticles are easily degraded in the cell and the products (Fe^{3+} ions) are used for cell metabolism [31–35].

In the present study, we demonstrate the role of iron oxide nanoparticles as nano-theranostics agents for cancer therapy. To this end, we express the intrinsic properties of these particles, their methods of preparation, and their applications in diagnostic, therapeutic, and nano-theranostics context.

---

[1]MNPs.
[2]MRI.

1.2 Iron Oxide Nanoparticles

MNPs have the potential to be applied in wide range of disciplines including magnetic fluids, biotechnology/biomedicine, biosensor, catalysis, data storage, MRI, and environmental remediation [36]. There exist several types of MNPs, ranging from pure metals (Fe, Co, Ni, and Mn) to metal oxides (Fe_3O_4, $\gamma\text{-}Fe_2O_3$), metal alloys (FePt, CoPt), and ferrites (MFe_2O_4, where M=Co, Cu, Ni, Mn, and Mg) that each could be used for a specific application [37].

Among the investigated MNPs, magnetite (Fe_3O_4) and maghemite ($\gamma\text{-}Fe_2O_3$) with cubic inverse spinel structure are the most applicable magnetic iron oxide that have attracted particular interest in nearly all above-mentioned fields and especially for different biomedical applications including enzyme encapsulation, cell separation and oligonucleotide identification, MRI, biosensor design, hyperthermia and targeted drug delivery due to its intrinsic properties such as appropriate size, high biocompatibility, low toxicity, and good magnetic properties. As for different applications, and especially biomedical application, it is critical to use nanoparticles which are chemically stable, uniform in size, and well dispersed in liquid media. These different characteristics of iron oxide nanoparticles such as size, structure, shape, and surface properties and their effects on magnetic properties should be investigated as well [36, 38, 39].

1.2.1 Properties of Magnetic Nanoparticles

1.2.1.1 Magnetic Behavior

Magnetite is considered as an important class of half-metallic materials, the molecular structure of which lets the electrons to hop between Fe^{2+} and Fe^{3+} ions in the octahedral sites at room temperature. Maghemite is the other type of iron oxide nanoparticles which can be easily synthesized from magnetite. Evidence showed that the existence of defects at the surface of both types of these particles could affected their magnetic properties [40, 41].

In order to study the magnetism of the particles, the hysteresis loop is usually referred to which is based on the relationship between magnetic field strength (H) and magnetization (M) of the particles (Fig. 1.1). The loop is generated by measuring the magnetic flux of a ferromagnetic material while the magnetizing force is changed. Saturation magnetization (M_s) is achieved when all the magnetic dipoles orientation of nanoparticle's domains aligned with the applied magnetic field. In the case of SPOINs, as ferromagnetic nanoparticles, by decreasing or removing the magnetic field, the orientation of some of domains is changed, so magnetization is decreased but does not reach zero. Retentivity magnetization (M_r) is the magnetic flux density that remains in the nanoparticles when the magnetizing force is removed.

By changing the direction of the magnetic field in the opposite direction, dipoles orientation is changed. In a certain point, the magnetization flux returns to zero

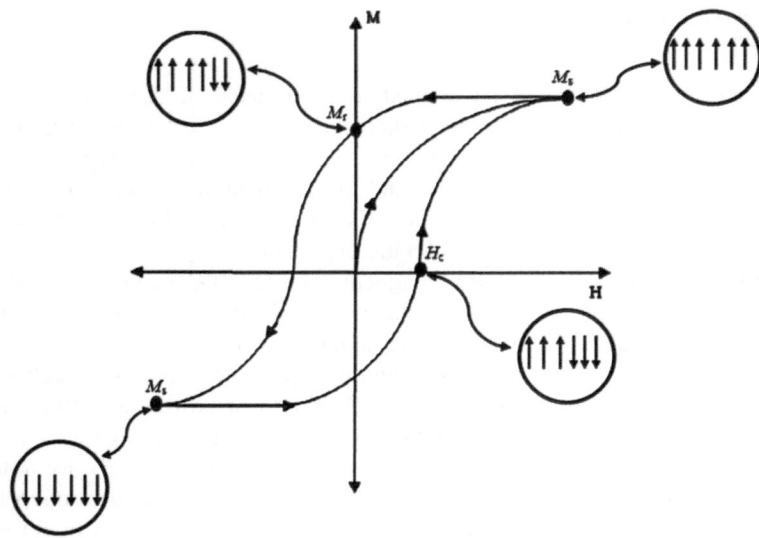

Fig. 1.1 Magnetization hysteresis loop

(H_c), the time in which the numbers of domains with opposite orientations are equal. After that, by increasing the magnetic field the magnetization is saturated again and this process will be repeated again and again in the presence of an alternating current (AC) magnetic field.

As mentioned by Frenkel and Dorfman for the first time, if the diameter of nanoparticles is decreased less than a critical particle size (<15 nm), MNPs exhibit superparamagnetic phenomena that dramatically change some of the magnetic properties. In fact, in the presence of an external magnetic field their magnetization can be saturated like other ferromagnetic materials, while their net magnetic moments are dropped to zero when the magnetic force is removed. Moreover, M_r and H_c points are deleted from the hysteresis loop of superpara MNPs due to their molecular structure which consists of a single magnetic domain [42–45]. Superparamagnetic iron oxide nanoparticles[3] propose important applications such as MRI, magnetically controlled drug carriers, and magnetic heterogeneous catalyst recovery [46, 47].

1.2.1.2   Size

Particle size is one of the most important characteristics of nanoparticles which could affect not only the properties of MNPs (as mentioned in the previous section), but also has an important role in their biomedical application [48, 49].

---

[3]SPIONs.

The specific surface area of nanoparticles (surface to mass ratio) has direct relationship with the size and has a dramatic impact on surface reactivity which could impress the body responds to nanoparticles and their distribution. Large particles are prone to be easily detected by the reticuloendothelial system (RES) and consequently be excluded from the blood stream [50, 51].

Size can also affect the mode of endocytosis, cellular uptake, and the efficiency of particle processing in the endocytic pathway. It is generally acknowledged that particles in the range of 10–30 nm could pass through the vessels and inter the cells through diffusion across plasma membrane or through membrane channels, while the larger particles are mainly carried into the cells by pinocytosis or phagocytosis [52, 53].

Method of preparation and preparation condition such as reaction time, temperature, ligand/precursor ratio as well as the solvents with different boiling points could also affect the particle size and size distribution, e.g., an increase in the temperature could lead to an increase in the particle size according to the Ostwald ripening law [54].

1.2.1.3 Charge

Surface charge plays an important role in nanoparticles biodistribution and cytotoxicity. While neutral particles has the lowest interactions with the plasma proteins (and less opsonization) which leads to an extended circulation time, high surface charge (positive or negative) enhances the phagocytosis process [55].

Positively charged particles attract proteins and immune system agents thus rapidly being cleared (within a few minutes) from the systemic circulation, where as strong negatively charged ones are uptaken by hepatic clearance system [56, 57].

Bare iron oxide nanoparticles are usually negatively charged due to the presence of limited numbers of hydroxyl groups on their surface. In the aqueous electrolyte solution, solid particles usually acquire a surface charge. This surface charge is usually presented onto certain types of nanoparticles (such as iron oxide and gold) to improve their stability and to prevent their aggregation in aqueous solution via the electrostatic repulsion [58]. Functionalization of MNPs by different polymers could introduce such charged groups on the surface of nanoparticles that not only prevent aggregation through increasing their water solubility but also affect their interactions with blood protein.

1.2.1.4 Surface Functionality and Colloidal Stability

Colloidal stability is one of the main requisites of nanoparticles in biomedical applications. Naked iron oxide particles have low stability in aqueous media and tend to aggregate due to the hydrophobic interactions. Aggregation causes a significant increase in the particles size and decreases their performance. The surface modification of MNPs by grafting stabilizing agents, such as biocompatible natural or synthetic polymers enhances their colloidal stability in a wide range of pH and in the presence of high amount of electrolytes [49, 59–62].

1.2.2 Methods of Preparation

Preparation method has direct effect on the main properties of MNPs such as size, shape, crystallinity, and magnetism. Parameters like temperature, pressure, pH, and molar ratio play the main role in this issue. Several approaches have been developed for the production of MNPs; each has its own advantages. Here we express some of the most popular methods with a brief explanation of their properties.

1.2.2.1 Copercipitation

This method is based on the synthesis of Fe_3O_4 from ferric chloride hexahydrate ($FeCl_3–6H_2O$) and ferrous chloride tetrahydrate ($FeCl_2–4H_2O$) as iron sources and ammonia as precipitator. It is the simplest and most common synthesis method. Moreover, it has high production yield and could be used to produce a broad range of nanoparticles with different sizes and shapes by adjusting pH, ionic strength, temperature, and other conditions of reaction. However, it has a limitation on the control of particle size distribution [63–65].

1.2.2.2 Sol-Gel

In this method, the base is hydration and condensation of precursors, leading to originating a sol of nanometric particles. Gel formation is achieved by further condensation as well as inorganic polymerization. In order to obtain the final crystalline structure, the as prepared gel is coupled by a heat treatment. The properties of the gel are attributed to the reaction conditions and the structure created within the sol stage [66–68].

1.2.2.3 Thermal Decomposition

This is a heating method which proceeds by decomposition of iron precursor (usually iron acetylacetonate (acac) or iron pentacarbonyl) at high temperature in the presence of solvent and stabilizer which leads to the production of monodispersed SPION with high crystallinity. By controlling the temperature, time of reaction and type, and ratio of solvent and precursor and their concentration, the size and morphology of nanoparticles could be controlled [69–71].

1.2.2.4 Polyol

It consists of an iron precursor and a polyol which acts as a solvent, reducing agent, and stabilizer. This method is based on preparing a suspension of the precursor and polyol and proceeds by heating the mixture until the polyol boiling point. Triethylene glycol (TREG) is one of the best polyols which is introduced by Cai and Wan that could produce uniform, non-agglomerate nanoparticles with narrow size distribution. Despite low production yield, this method is capable of producing narrow size distribution nanoparticles with enhanced magnetism due to the high crystallinity structure, which is soluble in the polar solvents due to the presence of polyol ligands on the surface of particles [72, 73].

Indeed, polyol is a specific type of thermal decomposition method that uses a liquid material (polyol) as both solvent and stabilizer simultaneously.

1.2.2.5 Sonolysis

Sonolysis is a class of thermal decomposition method, where cavities act as nanoreactors in which the required temperature for the reaction is produced. This process is based on sonolysis of organometallic precursors. In other words, the high temperature hot spot that is emerged through collapsing the cavities (made by sonication) lead to generation of iron oxide from ferrous salt [74–76].

1.2.2.6 Hydrothermal

This is another temperature-dependent method which is performed in the aqueous media under a high volume of pressure in reactors or autoclaves. In this process, wet chemical technology is used to produce highly crystalline iron oxide nanoparticles and the reaction conditions such as time, temperature, and solvent could affect the product's properties [77–80].

1.2.2.7 Microemulsion

Microemulsion is based on the dispersion of two immiscible liquids (water in oil or oil in water) in the presence of a surfactant. Nanoparticles are precipitated in the micelles formed in the hydrocarbon phase. Although the production yield of this process is low, it could be used to produce uniformly sized and crystalline SPIONs [36, 81, 82].

1.2.2.8 Green Synthesis

Biosynthesis or green synthesis is a new way for the synthesis of different nanoparticles in which a safe, cost-effective, environmental-friendly reagent is used to overcome the undesirable effects of toxic chemical materials that are used as solvent or capping agent in the process of synthesis. Here, nanocrystal iron oxide is synthesized in ambient conditions through the use of an iron metal salt (as iron precursor) and the animals or plants extracts (as solvent, reducing agent and also capping agent) or they can be extracted from the magnetosome of magnetotactic bacteria [83–85].

1.2.2.9 Other Methods

The above-mentioned methods are the most common techniques for iron oxide nanoparticles production. Aerosol, reverse micelle, flow injection, and electro-chemical method are some other methods with their own advantage and disadvantage that could be used for preparation of iron oxide nanoparticles.

1.3 Biomedical Applications

Iron oxide nanoparticles, due to their diverse and interesting properties have been used in a variety of disciplines for many years. The first use of magnetic materials in medicine is attributed to the internal applications of magnetite powder by the Egyptian physician and philosopher Avicenna in the tenth century. Recently, their applications in the biomedicine has been increased significantly [86]. The small size of SPIONs makes them an ideal candidate for drug and gene delivery system. Another medical application of SPIONs is hyperthermia treatment of cancer tissues, where SPIONs act as local overheating producers in response to an external magnetic field. Moreover, they can be used in bioseparation techniques for pollutant, cell labeling, protein purification, and tissue engineering. They also have applications in diagnosis field, which act as a contrast agent in MRI for better detection. Also in combination with other nanoparticles they could be used in other diagnosis techniques. Here we describe different biomedical applications of SPIONs in three subsections: biological applications, diagnosis, and therapy.

1.3.1 Biological Applications

1.3.1.1 Tissue Engineering

Tissue engineering, an interdisciplinary science which is based on the combination of cell biology, engineering, and medicine, has been developed to replace or regenerate damaged tissues. The main advantage of this technique is that it uses patient's autologous cells or stem cells and though reduces the risk of rejection [87]. Here, a three-dimensional scaffold is produced which is used for cells attachment and enhancement of their proliferation. Magnetic force-based tissue engineering (Mag-TE) is a novel technique that is used for this purpose in which magnetic nanodevices (e.g., magnetic gelatin nanoparticles, functionalized magnetic nanocarrier, MNP-loaded hydroxyapatite and collagen, magnetic cationic liposomes,[4] etc.) are applied to provide magnetoresponsive features [88–90]. Moreover, SPIONs could act as antimicrobial agents in the structure of scaffold. Indeed bacterial infection and biofilm generation is of the most challenging part of implanted medical devices. Incorporating SPIONs into the scaffold not only could provide an antimicrobial environment for scaffold, but also they could provide the ability of MR imaging during the treatment process [91–93].

MCLs entered the cells and then cells are adsorbed on the scaffold or on the targeted cell layer in the presence of magnetic field. Surface functionalization of MCLs by targeting agent and the strength of magnetic field has direct effect on the amount and depth of cell attachment [94–97].

3D cell culture technology or scaffold-free technology is an alternative way in tissue engineering in which MCL labeled cells are divided and grown in the presence of controlled magnetic forces. The geometry of the cell bulk could be operated by spatially controlling the magnetic field and scaffold-free portions of tissues in a variety of shapes could be achieved. Skin, liver, and muscle tissues are some examples build by this technique [98–100].

1.3.1.2 Magnetic Separation

One of the most useful technological applications of iron oxide nanoparticles is magnetic separation, which is successfully applied in broad aspects of biological and biomedical researches including protein purification, toxin decorporation, virus and bacterial separation, enzyme fixation, and cell labeling. It is a high sensitive technique and could separate low number of targeted agents [101–103]. It could be combined with other detection techniques and therefore enhance the accuracy and sensitivity of the assay. Magnetic enzyme linked immunosorbent assay is an example in which the fluorescent enzymes are used to determine the concentration of the materials optically [104]. Surface functionalization of MNPs with polymers, ligands, or suitable surfactant could improve their separation properties due to the selective receptor–ligand interactions occurred [105].

In comparison with other conventional techniques, magnetic separation could be more applicable due to its good adaptation, ability to work without need of pretreatment process, easy, fast, and economical methodology with reusable sorbent [106].

There are two approaches for magnetic separation purposes; conventional method which is used inlaboratory and contains direct and indirect modes (Fig. 1.2), and other methods which are used for industrial scale. In this context it

---

[4]MCLs.

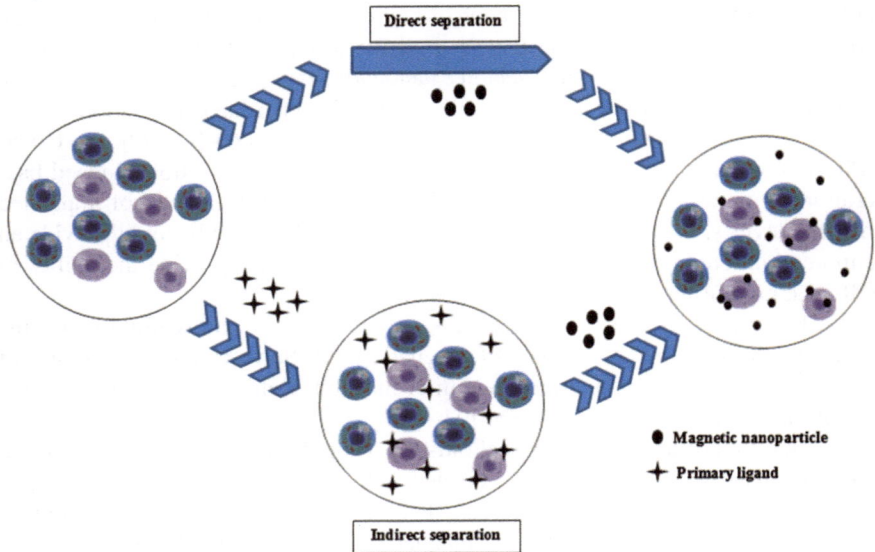

Fig. 1.2 Conventional methods of magnetic separation: direct and indirect

can be note tothe magnetically stabilized fluidized beds (MSFB) which is a continuous separation procedure for biological products and also biocompatible two phasesystems which are used for separation of cells, subcellular organelles and biologically active compounds [107, 108].

In the direct mode, separation is based on the attachment of magnetic affinity particles to the targeted material and then collecting them through foreign magnetic field, while indirect method is started by insertion of free affinity ligands to the targeted compounds and then this complex is captured by magnetic particles through affinity interactions [109]. Direct method is easier and faster than the other and needs fewer amounts of ligands however indirect method is more efficient and sensitive especially in the case of targeted compound with poor affinity [110, 111].

1.3.1.3   Toxin Decorporation

Nanoparticles are promising materials for collection of deleterious components such as radioactive materials, uranyl ions, metal ions, and drugs from environment and living organism due to their high specific surface area. For biodetoxification of blood and tissues, for example, from over dose of drug, nanocarriers should have some critical properties like long circulation time (to extract sufficient amount of toxic drugs from the blood and surrounded tissues), high stable detoxification capacity (to prevent rapid release of the trapped drug back), and appropriate surface functional groups (to increase the circulation time and drug capturing capacity) [112].

Magnetic nanoparticles are one of these nanocarriers which can act as detoxifiers in different forms, e.g., polymer-based magnetic nanospheres, magnetic beads, and surface-functionalized magnetic particles. According to literature, surface functionalization of nanoparticles with different modalities such as tetraethyl-3-aminopropane-1,1-bisphosphonate (BP), biocompatible polymers like polyethylene glycol and its copolymer with polylactic acid could accelerate toxin trapping process [113–115].

1.3.1.4 Virus and Bacterial Separation

Immunomagnetic nanoparticles are MNPs which are functionalized with antibodies designed for separation of bacteria from biological environment. Attachment of cell-specific ligands on the surface of MNPs is another strategy for exclusive separation of viruses and bacteria. Due to the use of these functionalizing agents, the detection and separation procedure is done in a high level of accuracy and specificity. Moreover, the sensitivity of this process is greater than other strategies which could detect small number of pathogens in a short time [111, 116]. The magnetic surface-enhanced Raman spectroscopy (SERS), MRI, and miniaturized NMR system are techniques that could be used for detection and monitoring of this process. MNPs coupled with virus-specific globulin proteins were used for adsorption of hepatitis B viral (HBV) and hepatitis C viral (HCV) particles present in sera. *E. coli, Bacillus anthracis, Mycobacterium avium, Mycobacterium tuberculosis,* and *Staphylococcus aureus* are bacterial samples which have been separated through surface functionalized magnetic nanoparticles [117–121].

1.3.1.5 Protein and Nucleic Acid Separation

Magnetic separation is an attractive method for selection and purification of the intended protein or nucleic acid (DNA/RNA) in a cheap, easy, short time, and scalable manner without any sample pretreatment process. The intrinsic properties of nanoparticles such as good dispersity and high surface to volume ratio and the structural changes of the adsorbed protein, cause to increase the binding capacity and specificity of this method [102, 122, 123]. Surface functionalization of MNPs is the method used for accelerating the connection between nanoparticles and peptides. The use of MNPs functionalized with ligands bearing Ni^{2+}-chelating species such as nitrilotriacetic acid (NTA) for the separation of histidine-tag (his-tag) proteins is one of the most popular protein separation strategies. Graphene-functionalized magnetic silica, fullerene-functionalized magnetic silica microsphere, MNPs functionalized with specific peptides for antibody separation, and magnetic molecularly imprinted polymers (MMIPs) for the selective enrichment of proteins are other sample strategies [107, 124–127].

In the case of nucleic acid separation, which is an important tool for molecular biology, the hybridization of targeted nucleic acid with oligonucleotide grafted on

MNPs plays a critical role. This process leads to isolation of an oligonucleotide which could be amplified by polymerase chain reaction (PCR) and could be used for sequencing assay or could be labeled for other detection processes [128–130].

1.3.1.6 Enzyme Immobilization

Immobilization is a cost-effective, time-consuming procedure which is suitable for promoting different properties of enzymes including the optimization of enzyme's activity, its reusability, storage, and operational conditions stability (thermal and pH) and also provides the ability for use in continuous operating mode and facilitates its separation from the reaction mixture. Magnetic nanoparticles are good candidate for immobilization since they could be quickly separated from the digestion environment in the presence of magnetic field. Immobilization process on MNPs could be performed through either covalent bonding, which is the most commonly used technique with surface functionalization of MNPs and has advantages like higher thermal and structural stability or physical adsorption which is dependent on hydrogen bonds, ionic interactions, hydrophobic interactions, van der Waals forces, etc., as binding forces without need of reagent or pretreatment steps. Moreover, enzyme-immobilized magnetic materials could be coupled with a certain digestion techniques like microwave, microfluidic, and chip to reduce its digestion time to minutes or seconds, enhance its sensitivity and promote the efficiency of the digestion reaction [107, 131–134].

1.3.1.7 Cell Labeling and Separation

Cell labeling with MNPs is a novel technique for monitoring and tracking the cells inside the body of living organism via MRI. Challenge points in the cell labeling process are (i) achieving the high level of labeling which is attributed to the amount of SPIONs uptake by the cells and could be increased by targeting the nanoparticles and (ii) confirming that the cell viability and integrity is not influenced through labeling [135, 136].

There are varieties of methods for cell labeling with SPIONs which are used according to the specific purpose. They are categorized into three fundamental classes: (i) in vitro approaches (e.g., through endocytosis, transfection agents, magnetofection, electroporation), (ii) in vivo cell labeling by reticuloendothelial system (RES) through systemic application, and (iii) receptor-mediated binding and internalization of SPIONs by targeted cells (e.g., targeted labeling and imaging) [137].

One of the applications of cell labeling is stem cells tracking and monitoring which are used for cell transplantation therapy purposes (Fig. 1.3). Stem cell transplantation could be broadly applied in regenerative medicine for treatment of heart failure, vascular injury, ventricular disfunction, and numerous diseases such as myocardial infarction, neurologic diseases, and cancer [138–140]. Isolation of

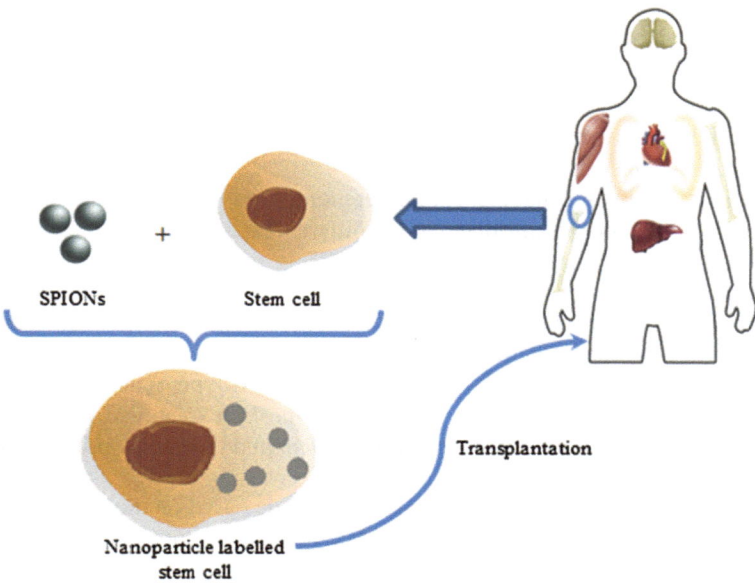

Fig. 1.3 Stem cell labeling with magnetic nanoparticles

cancer cells from the blood and other tissues is another application of SPION-tagged cells that require surface functionalization of SPIONs with targeting ligands like antibodies, folate, aptamers, etc. For example, conjugation of anti-CD34 antibodies to the surface of SPIONs could allow targeting of labeled nanoparticles toward acute leukemia cells. This process is designed based on immunomagnetic separation and could be used for detection of circulating tumor cells[5] and also enrichment of stem cells [141–144].

1.3.2 Theranostics and Nano-Theranostics Applications of SPIONs

1.3.2.1 Theranostics and Nano-Theranostics

Theranostics or theragnostics is defined as the fusion of diagnostics and therapy and can be classified into three categories, therapy followed by diagnosis, diagnosis followed by therapy, and the concomitant use of therapeutics and diagnostics. Theranostics was introduced by Funkhouser as any "material that combines the modalities of therapy and diagnostic imaging" into a single package, in 2002. The

---

[5]CTCs.

aim of designing theranostics agents is to detect and treat disease at their early stage, to monitor the efficiency of treatment process, and to reduce the waste of time for diagnosis and therapy [145–148]. Real-time visualization of nanodrug carrier biodistributions, drug release processes, and therapeutic responses can provide critical information needed for dynamically optimizing treatment operations in a personalized manner in real time [149].

Now it is well known that there are different responds to a particular treatment in different patients which is attributed to the differences in their genomics and results in the generation of the new era in the medicine that is named as personalized medicine and can be defined as "the right drug for the right person administered at the right time." It is a beneficial therapeutic approach especially in serious diseases like cancer, AIDS, and atherosclerosis and its cerebrovascular and cardiovascular appearances. The use of theranostic (and its improved type, nano-theranostics) in this field can empower physicians to perform the best treatment plan based on monitoring the personalized response of the patient and therefore optimize the dose of drugs and reduce the side effects [150–153].

Nano-theranostics or theranostics nanomedicine is based on the accumulation of diagnosis and therapeutic agents into nanocarriers such as liposomes, micelles, carbon nanotubes, nanoparticles, polymer-based nanomaterials, and so on for medical applications. The advantage of nanoparticles in faster penetration to the various parts of body and the possibility of guiding them to the targeted tissue through attachment of targeting agents make them ideal cases that improve traditional application of theranostics agents [154, 155]. The imaging part of the nanotheranostics is based on the use of fluorescent dyes like quantum dots (for optical imaging), magnetic nanoparticles, i.e., SPIONs (for MRI), radionuclides (as nuclear imaging agents), and heavy elements, e.g., iodine [for computed tomography (CT)] and the other part includes different types of drugs, proteins, or aptamers which are designed and selected according to the special disease. The interesting matter about nano-theranostics is that some of the nanocarriers have intrinsic imaging and/or therapeutic property; in fact they are applied as self-theranostics platforms [156, 157].

SPIONs based nanoplatforms are such a nano-theranostics that used MRI as their monitoring strategy. Moreover, these nanocarriers can be coupled with other diagnosis strategies turning to the synthesis of more sensitive and accurate nano-theranostics device. The therapeutic property of these carriers is classified into two categories: intrinsic therapeutic property of SPIONs that is attributed to their magnetic property and is known as hyperthermia and magnetic-based separation. In the other case, SPIONs act as carriers for therapeutic agents (drug/genes or other nanoparticles with therapeutic properties) (Fig. 1.4).

1.3.2.2 Diagnosis

In general, diagnosis is a critical step in medical researches which affects the treatment process, and not only includes the early detection of disease, but also covers the treatment and recovery processes. Imaging methods play the main role in

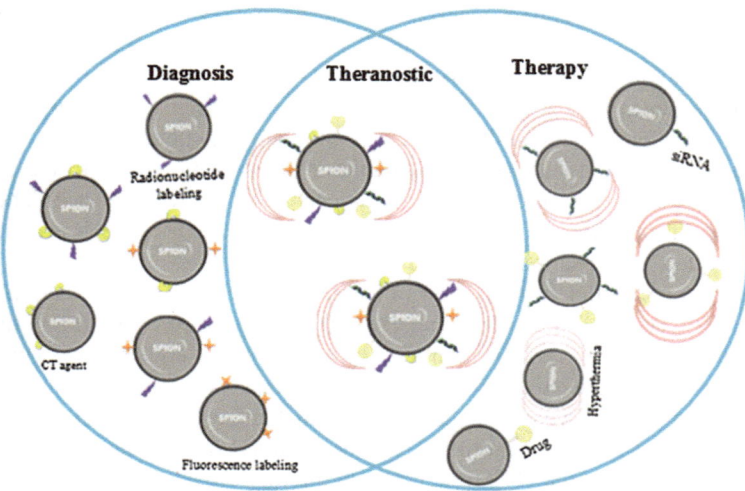

Fig. 1.4 SPIONs as nano-theranostics agents

this context. MRI, CT, positron emission tomography (PET), single-photon emission computed tomography (SPECT), ultrasound (US) imaging, and optical imaging are some of common imaging techniques which are used for this purpose [158–163].

The application of nanoparticles in imaging techniques has provided the possibility of simultaneous application of two or more imaging methods. SPIONs are ideal candidates as contrast agents in MRI. Based on this principle, SPIONs could be applied in format of sensors, separation tools, or biomedical devices for detecting and monitoring the target agents [164].

In this section, we describe the principles of MRI, effects of SPIONs on MR imaging improvement, and different applications of SPIONs based on MRI application.

Magnetic Resonance Imaging (MRI): Principles and Applications

MRI is a noninvasive powerful diagnostic modality which is based on the principles of nuclear magnetic resonance[6] providing high-resolution anatomical images from inside the body. Indeed, images are formed based on detecting the proton relaxation in the presence of an external magnetic field [165–167]. MRI has several advantages over other imaging techniques including high spatial resolution, enhanced soft

---

[6]NMR.

tissue contrast, and excellent anatomic detail. Moreover, in comparison to other imaging techniques such as CT and PET, it is more safe because of lack of the concern of radiation exposure [168, 169].

In the presence of a strong magnetic field, the hydrogen nuclear spins are oriented in parallel or antiparallel direction of magnetic field. Using a resonant radiofrequency irradiation, which is capable of transferring energy to the protons, the numbers of excited protons with high energy state are increased. Then, the pulsing field turns off and magnetic moments of protons return to their original state that is entitled as relaxation [170, 171].

There are two different relaxation processes: longitudinal magnetization recovery (T1-recovery) and transverse magnetization decay (T2-decay). T1 is the time taken for longitudinal magnetization to recover 63% of the equilibrium, while T2 is the time needed for the exponential decay of the transverse magnetization to 37% of its initial magnitude. Two critical parameters which affected the signal intensity and image contrast are repetition time (TR, time between radiofrequency pulse replication) and the echo time (TE, time between the radiofrequency pulse and the first signal measurement). In T1-weighted image, both TR (250–700 ms) and TE (10–25 ms) are selected as short time, while for T2 state, images are generated by long TR (>2000 ms) and TE (TE > 60 ms). Different tissues have shown different contrasts. Tissues with short T1 cause brightness in the MRI images and tissues with short T2 lead to a darkness in imaging [172–174].

The intrinsic T1 and T2 relaxation properties of most tissues are not sufficient and lead to a reduction in the image quality. Exogenous contrast agent materials are used in order to enhance the visibility of the images by altering the relaxation time. Relaxivity (r1 and r2) is the parameter which have affected the efficiency of contrast agent and is defined as the change occurs in the relaxation rate ($R1 = 1/T1$ and $R2 = 1/T2$ in units of s^{-1}) of solvent water protons in the presence of contrast agent [175].

Paramagnetic materials, especially gadolinium, are the most common contrast agents which are generally used. Gadolinium is a (T1) widely used contrast agent that increases the signal intensity by decreasing T1 relaxation time and produce brighter (T1-weighted) images [176]. However, its low sensitivity, short blood circulation, and possible toxicity lead to the introduction of novel contrast materials [177]. SPIONs are one of the most suitable cases for this purpose that has recently been proposed as T2 negative contrast agent. The interactions between spin of water protons and SPIONs cause change in the spin–spin relaxation of water molecules around the nanoparticles and thus reduce the T2 relaxation time and generate a darker (T2-weighted) image [178, 179]. Moreover, SPIONs can act as T1 contrast agents if their size reduces to a critical level which is due to the powerful magnetic property and large surface area for water diffusion [180–182]. SPIONs have advantages compared with conventional contrast agent including higher relaxivity, more sensitivity, appropriate blood half-life, good biocompatibility and biodegradability [183].

Application of SPIONs in MRI makes it a useful diagnostic agent which is utilized in a wide range of field. Magnetic separation that mentioned earlier is one of these applications in which magnetic nanoparticles act as separation agent and MRI contrast agent simultaneously and provide the ability to isolate different factors such as nucleic acids, proteins, bacteria, viruses, and even polluting agents. In other words, SPION acts as a nanosensor in which detection process is visualized through changing in the spin–spin relaxation times of water molecules. Surface modification of nanoparticles enhances the detection of targeted molecules [164, 184, 185].

Another application of SPIONs is diagnosis of inflammatory and neurodegenerative disease since early detection of such disease is important for successful treatment. Attachment of endothelial cell adhesion molecules like selectins to the surface of SPIONs could target these nanoparticles toward the cells with overexpression of these compounds which are the characteristic of early stages of atherosclerosis. Moreover, γ-Fe_2O_3 nanoparticles were used for identification efficiency of the drugs which was used against plaque inflammation. Neuroinflammation disease (e.g., multiple sclerosis[7]) could also be monitored by SPIONs through enhancing the detection process in comparison to the cases which used gadolinium in MR imaging. Alzheimer's disease could also be detected through the conjugation of antibodies on the surface of SPIONs against the amyloid fibrils of the amyloid plaques [186–191].

Cancer is another class of disease which could be detected using SPION-based MRI. Surface functionalization of SPIONs with cancer's specific ligands, leads to identify and connect to the tumor tissue and enables in vivo tissue imaging during treatment process. As noted above, early detection especially in the first stage of cancer plays the key role in treatment. Moreover, these SPIONs could act as carriers of therapeutic agents to accelerate the healing process. These drug delivery systems are named as theranostic agents which proposed a new application field in medicine which will be explained later.

Multimodal Imaging

The next generation of MRI-based contrast materials consist of core–shell structure which provides the possibility of using two different imaging techniques simultaneously (multimodal imaging) improving the sensitivity and accuracy of detection (Fig. 1.5). This includes:

1. MR/Optical imaging: Here, SPION core could be attached directly to the fluorophores or be coated with a biocompatible shell (like dextran, polyethylene glycol,[8] silica, etc.) which is functionalized with a fluorescence probe. Cy5, rhodamine B, and fluorescein isothiocyanate[9] are the most popular materials

---

[7]MS.
[8]PEG.
[9]FITC.

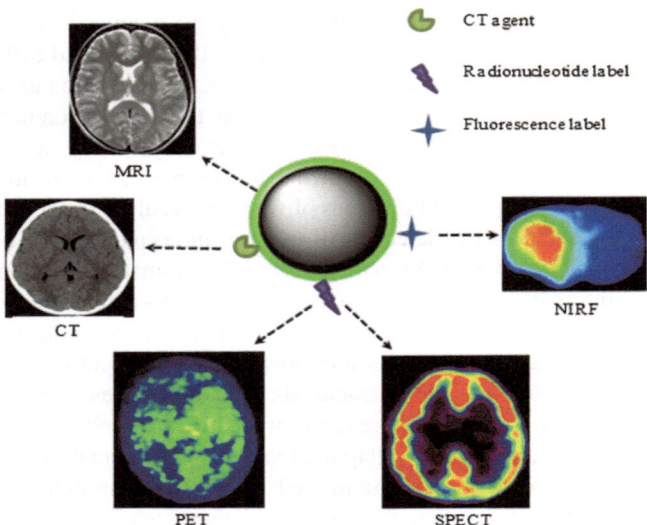

Fig. 1.5 Multimodal imaging based on SPION

which are used as optical agents. This new combined probe has the sensitivity of optical imaging and the resolution property of MRI simultaneously [192–194].

2. MR/PET imaging: PET is an extraordinarily sensitive imaging modality with poor resolution that constructs images using the signals emitted from radioactive tracer (11C, 18F, 64Cu, 68Ga, and 124I). In this case, radionuclide is grafted on to the polymer-coated SPION. This provides a quantitative, phenomenal, high-resolution method with no penetration limit [195, 196].

3. MR/CT imaging: CT is a common medical imaging that uses computer-processed X-rays for producing images. In comparison to the MRI, this could prepare high temporal resolution and could provide images from various organs, but it has limitations for soft tissue which is due to its low sensitivity. Therefore, the combination of these two modalities could cover their defects. For this purpose, iodine as the most routine CT imaging agent, and noble metals (gold and silver) are used. These agents could be attached directly to the surface of SPION or could be used as a coating on the surface of SPION or could be considered as the heterostructured nanoparticles [197–199].

4. MR/US imaging: Diagnostic sonography is a cost-effective, highly safe, real-time imaging technique that uses the rate differences of the US passage through different tissues for imaging construction. However, it could be used only for superficial and echogenic tissues due to the limitation of penetration. Application of microbubbles, as US contrast agents, which are functionalized with SPION provide strong contrast in MRI and US [168, 200, 201].

1.3.2.3 Therapy

Therapy is one of the three compartments of medication in which an external factor is used to promote the immune system operation to return the health state. This external factor could be chemical drugs, which are commonly used for variety of diseases, different types of beams, and even artificial limb. Nanotechnology as a multidisciplinary field could be applied in various areas of medicine. Indeed, it emerged as a new field in medical science which is named nanomedicine and could be applied not only for diagnostic applications, but also provided the ability to disease prevention and treatment. In the field of therapy, it could be helpful by introduction of new approach, preparation of a wide range of drug delivery systems, and providing conditions for the simultaneous application of two or more treatment manner. Depending on the nanomaterial that has been used, nanomedicine could be applied for treatment of various diseases, from inflammations (e.g., diabetes, Alzheimer, MS, etc.) to different types of cancer. SPIONs are one of the most widely used class of nanoparticles with different intrinsic therapeutic capabilities which made them appropriate tools for application in a variety of treatment methods, including hyperthermia, photothermal therapy, photodynamic therapy, tissue engineering, combination therapy, and especially drug and gene delivery [202–205].

Hyperthermia

Overheating or hyperthermia is defined as treatment of disease with the aim of the heat (Fig. 1.6). Although the first application of hyperthermia is gone back to the last centuries, its modern clinical applications started from 1950s. Gilchrist et al. were the first who used magnetic nanoparticles (γ-Fe$_2$O$_3$) to produce heat in the

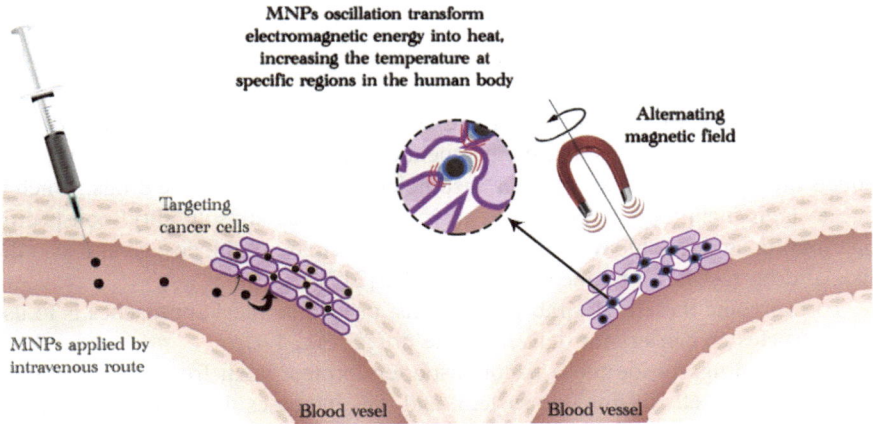

Fig. 1.6 Destruction of tumor tissue with magnetic hyperthermia

presence of magnetic field in 1957 and since then different types of magnetic nanoparticles were used as heat producer in hyperthermia. Although there are different approaches to produce heat, e.g., microwave, radiofrequency, US, utilizing MNPs is preferred due to their ability of controlling the temperature switching and more importantly the potential of centralization of MNPs in the targeted tissue which in turn increases the efficiency of hyperthermia and reduces the heating side effects on the surrounding tissues. Hyperthermia is used for treatment of different types of disease such as gonococcal infection, blood coagulation in small vessels, HIV infection, and especially cancer treatment, which constituted the majority of researches in the field of hyperthermia since cancerous cells show more sensitivity to the heat induction in comparison to the healthy one. Indeed, today hyperthermia is the fifth common method of cancer treatment [206–209].

Based on the amount of heat generated, there are two kinds of heating treatments: induction heating of cells between 41 and 46 °C, which is usually known as hyperthermia leading to DNA damage, protein denaturation, and cell apoptosis due to the thermal stress, and thermo ablation (also named as hyperthermia) which is performed at higher temperatures, up to 56 °C, and results into necrosis, carbonization, or coagulation of the targeted tissue [210–214].

The generated heat is attributed to the relaxation processes and hysteresis losses of MNPs which are impressed by a foreign alternating current (AC). Among them, SPIONs with no hysteresis loop could also be used to generate heat. Their small size accelerates the rate of cell absorption, and their surface functionalized groups deliver them to the targeted tissues. Brownian rotation which is due to the rotation of the particles is one of the reasons for heat generation in both types of nanoparticles. Since SPIONs are single-domain particles, the hysteresis loss is not considered for them and the heat generation is due to the energy which is provided by the AC magnetic field inducing rotation to the magnetic moment of particles. Returning to the relaxation orientation leads the trapped energy to release as heat, the phenomena which is recognized as Ne'el relaxation [210, 215, 216].

Drug and Gene Delivery

The overall objective of the design and construction of nanocarriers is to deliver sufficient amount of drugs and biotherapeutic to the targeted site without any side effects on the healthy organs. In fact, insufficient effectiveness of the drugs, which is due to their inappropriate properties such as poor aqueous solubility, nonspecific distribution, and low bioavailability, leads to an increase in the dosage and also the risk of drug resistance by the offending agent [217].

To overcome these undesirable conditions, one of the ideal approaches is to use nanoparticles as carriers for delivering the drugs (Fig. 1.7).

Loading drugs inside these nanotransporters protect them from recognition by the phagocytic cells of immune system, and thus increases their blood circulation, delivers them to the targeted tissue with the least impression on healthy tissues. Thus, carrier-mediated drug delivery has the potential of releasing drug inside the

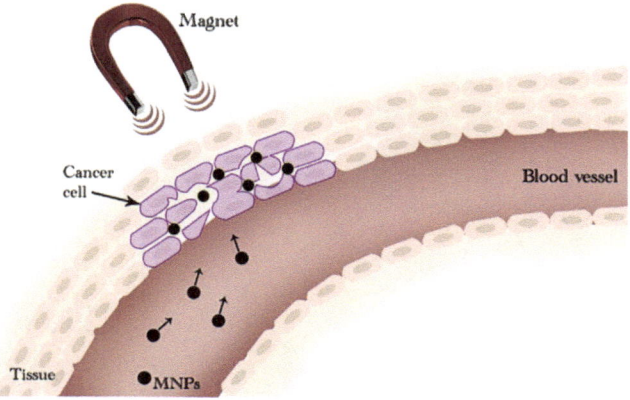

Fig. 1.7 Drug delivery system based on SPIONs

cells which subsequently improves the drug's efficiency. Some of the nanoparticles have therapeutic properties themselves and can be used alone for treatment of disease or in combination with other therapeutic methods enhancing the efficiency of treatment. In this context, Ag and Fe nanoparticles could be noted which could induce cytotoxicity effects when they are in the form of ions. Combination therapy is the preferred way for treatment of incurable diseases like different types of cancer, in which the treatment effects of combined approaches are equal or higher (named as additive and synergistic effect, respectively) than the effect of each approach separately.

As an in vivo vehicle, the physicochemical properties of nanoparticles should be considered before production. These properties include size and size distribution, stability, and surface functionality. Monodispersed nanoparticles with the size range under 100 nm are suitable for biomedical applications. Surface functionalization with biocompatible polymers increases the drug loading efficiency, the water solubility, and the possibility for attachment of targeting/tracing moieties (Fig. 1.8) [218–220].

Targeting Approaches

Targeting nanoparticles for a specific tissue could increase the efficiency of drugs and reduce the required drug dosage. There are two traditional approaches for targeting nanoparticles (Fig. 1.9):

1. Passive targeting: This is the initial driving force for delivering the nanoparticles to the target tissue which is based on the size of nanoparticles and intrinsic properties of tissue which is known as the enhanced permeability and retention[10]

---

[10]EPR.

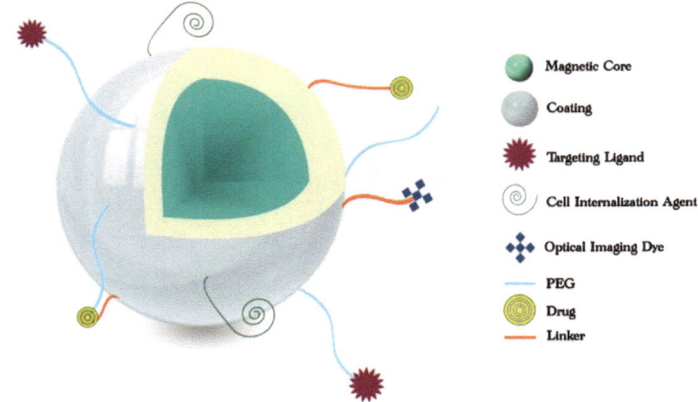

Fig. 1.8 Schematic of SPION with multifunctional decoration

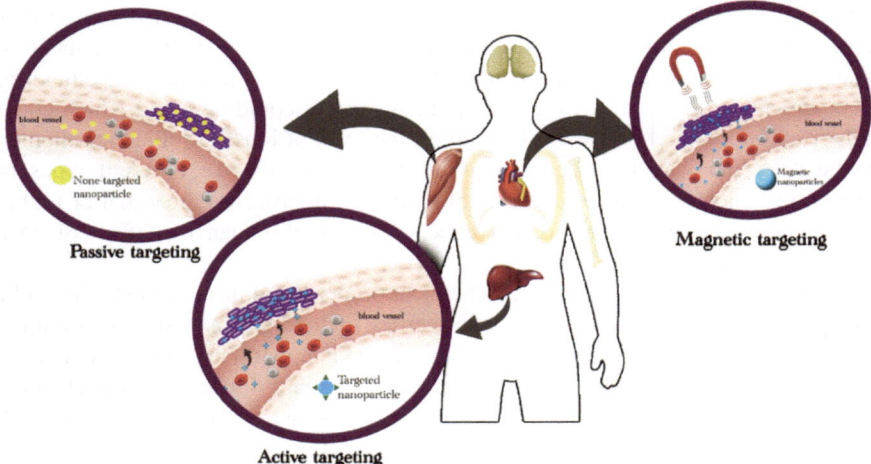

Fig. 1.9 Different targeting approaches with SPIONs

effect. In some diseases like cancer and inflammation, changes in the intercellular distance enhance the permeability of the vessels which leads to an increase in the amount of materials that penetrate from them; while the retention of the materials to the blood stream is limited, the result is the accumulation of the nanoparticles in the tissue [221, 222].

2. Active targeting: This approach is based on employment of specific targeting ligands which are attached on the surface of nanoparticles and accelerate the cell accumulation of nanoparticles. So far, various types of targeting moieties have been used among them are folic acid, aptamers, protein, and peptides like antibodies and RGD peptide (L-arginine, glycine, and L-aspartic acid)

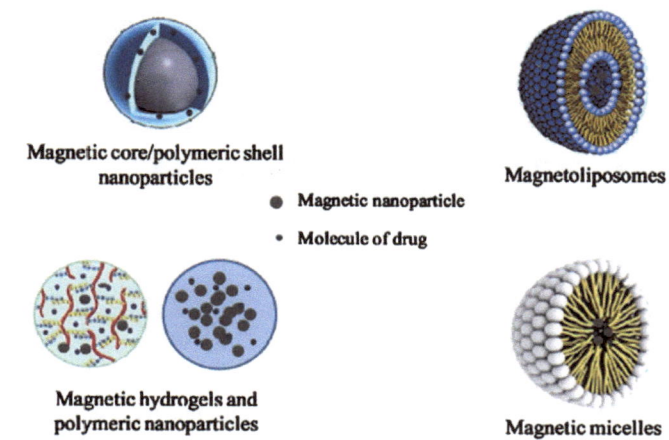

Magnetic core/polymeric shell nanoparticles

Magnetoliposomes

● Magnetic nanoparticle

• Molecule of drug

Magnetic hydrogels and polymeric nanoparticles

Magnetic micelles

Fig. 1.10 Different types of magnetic-based nanoparticles

[223–225]. Magnetic targeting in the presence of magnetic field is another approach that could be categorized in the batch of active targeting. This makes iron oxide nanoparticles an ideal candidate as drug delivery vehicle [226].

In conclusion, after MRI, drug delivery is the most important field of application of SPIONs in biomedicine, phenomena that was started in 1963 by Meyer. The small particle size and the possibility of surface engineering are the other suitable properties of SPIONs in drug delivery applications. Therapeutic agents could be attached directly to the surface of SPIONs or be floated in the space surrounded by the coating agent [227].

Surface Functionalization

As mentioned previously, it is necessary for SPIONs to be treated with different functionalization agents due to the intrinsic properties of these particles (Fig. 1.10). These surfaces include polymeric coating, magnetic nanocomposite, hydrogels, micelles, liposomes, and microspheres which can improve their loading efficiency and biocompatibility and provide the possibility of attachment of targeting agents leading to multimodal targeting systems. The process of drug release from these carriers is based on the corrosion, leakage, shrinking, and intracellular degradation [228, 229].

Some of the most popular natural and synthetic polymers that are used for this purpose are chitosan, dextran, polylactic acid,[11] polyglycolic acid,[12] polyvinyl

---

[11]PLA.
[12]PGA.

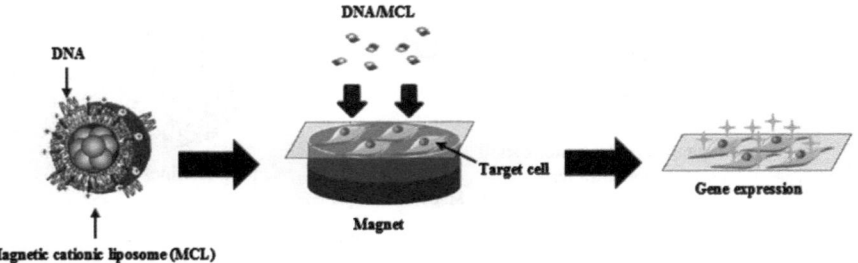

Fig. 1.11 MCL magnetofection

alcohol,[13] polyethylene glycol, polyglycerol, and so on. They could be applied in two forms of liner and dendritic shape, or be combined with each other to form copolymer (poly lactic glycolic acid[14]). Responsive polymers, like poly(N-iso-propylacrylamide)[15] and poly(N-vinylcaprolactam)[16] are the new generation of polymers with a phase transition point which are sensitive to the changes occurred in surrounding conditions such as pH, ionic strength, or temperature. Smart drug delivery systems are the class of carriers which are made based on these responsive polymers [230–236].

Liposomes also can be used for trapping the SPIONs. Moreover, their bilayered geometry makes it possible to load multiple drugs and introduce them as multidrug delivery systems for the treatment of multidrug resistant tumors [237]. In this regard, amphiphilic polymers or copolymers (like PEG and PG) that have lipophilic and hydrophilic compartments for loading hydrophobic and hydrophilic drugs simultaneously are of great interest.

Antibiotics, antibacterial, and anti-inflammation drugs are the most popular therapeutic agents which could be transferred by the SPIONs. Antibacterial properties of SPIONs in combination with conjugated bactericides like antibiotics provide a multidrug factor that simplify interactions between bacteria and bactericides and enhance the healing process [238]. Anticancer drugs are another class of therapeutic agents that can be carried by SPIONs based drug delivery systems. In fact, the hydrophobic nature of most of these drugs and their harmful effects on normal tissues along with the ability of SPIONs based drug delivery systems for loading these drugs, have attracted numerous researches to this field [231, 239, 240].

SPIONs, as a platform, could be used for delivering therapeutic genes or nucleic acids, the phenomenon which is known as magnetofection and was introduced by Kuehnle in 1994 (Fig. 1.11). DNA, small interfering ribonucleic acid[17] or antisense

---

[13]PVA.

[14]PLGA.

[15]PNIPAAM.

[16]PVCL.

[17]siRNA.

oligonucleotides are conjugated to the SPIONs through electrostatic interactions between positive charge of cationic-coated SPIONs and negative charge of nucleic acid and thus could be guided through the external magnetic field to the targeted cells [241–243].

Other Therapy

Delivering the stem cells to a targeted tissue or their transplantation using SPIONs as labeling agents for cells is another therapeutical application of SPIONs. SPIONs inside or on the surface of cells, not only act as carrier for stem cells, but also make it possible to monitor the fate of therapeutic process [244].

Photothermal therapy[18] is a therapeutic approach for cancer treatment which is based on stimulation of heat by nanoparticles that are influenced with near-infrared[19] laser light (photothermal absorber[20]). SPIONs based PTT is classified into two categories: typical approach is based on modification of the surface of SPIONs with PTA agents. Coating with gold nanoparticles is the most common PTA that is used for this purpose. Recently, highly concentrated SPIONs and clustered Fe_3O_4 nanoparticles are introduced as new PTA agents (Fig. 1.12). Indeed, PTT with SPIONs can be classified as a subcategory of hyperthermia in which NIR is used instead of alternating magnetic field[21] for heat producing process [32, 245, 246].

Surface functionalization of magnetic nanoparticles makes it possible to use these nanoparticles in combination therapy modalities in which MNPs act as targeting agent as well as chemotherapeutic carrier. Based on the suggested therapeutic approach, different agents could be coated on the SPIONs, for example, attachment of photosensitizer like porphyrins or methylene blue make it possible to use these particles in photodynamic therapy,[22] which is based on the production of reactive oxygen species[23] through the effect of light on the photosensitizer [247, 248]. Sonodynamic therapy[24] is another application, in which SPIONs could act as a sonosensitizer that enhance the therapeutic effects of ultrasonic waves [249, 250].

It should be noted that in all of these therapeutic applications, SPIONs act as diagnosis agent that provides the possibility of tracing therapeutic effect, the phenomenon that introduced SPIONs as theranostic agents and will be discussed in the next section.

---

[18]PTT.
[19]NIR.
[20]PTA.
[21]AMF.
[22]PDT.
[23]ROS.
[24]SDT.

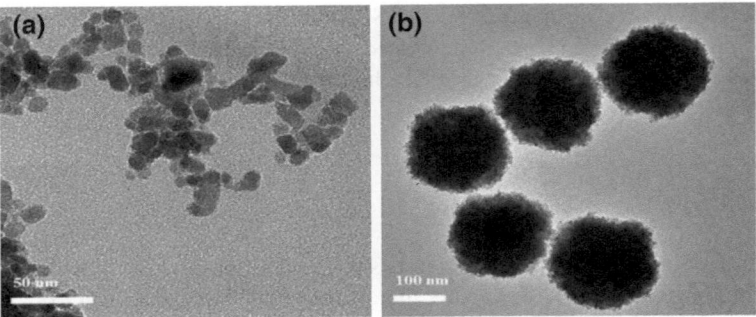

Fig. 1.12 TEM images of **a** Fe₃O₄ NPs and **b** clustered magnetic Fe₃O₄ NPs (Reprinted with permission from Ref. [32])

1.3.2.4 SPIONs Based Nano-Theranostics for Cancer Therapy

Today SPION is the only nanoparticle that has FDA approval for application in the body. Based on this, some commercial types of SPION have been propagated including Feridex or ferum oxides as imaging agents for liver lesions; Combidex or ferumoxtran-10 (Sinerem®, Guerbert) for imaging of "hidden" prostate cancer lymph node metastases; and Feraheme or ferumoxytol for treating iron deficiency anemia in chronic kidney diseases [251].

Till now a wide range of researches have been conducted in which different modifications are used in order to introduce the best one with improved properties like biocompatibility, hydrophilicity, lack of immune system activation, high drug loading capacity, and controlled drug release. Moreover, this coating material should have no/less effect on magnetic properties of SPIONs. Phospholipids (entitled as magnetoliposomes), different proteins, ligands, and polymeric materials are some of these stabilizers that have been used with SPIONs.

Multifunctional nanoparticles with the ability of nano-theranostics applications have been proposed by different researchers. Yang et al. prepared SPIONs decorated with poly(aspartic acid) (as a biodegradable polymer) and introduced it as a carrier for DOX as well as a T2 contrast agent for MRI [252]. For a similar application, Xu et al. used nanocomposite of SPIONs with a block copolymer for DOX delivery and introduced it for image-guided therapy [253].

Hyperbranched and dendrimeric polymers are also good platforms due to their high drug loading capacity. Hyperbranched polyglycerol[25] as a highly hydrophilic and biocompatible polymer grafted to SPIONs for delivering curcumin to cancer cells is such a theranostic nanoplatform which is introduced by Jahandar et al. [254].

---

[25]HPG.

In another study, Nasongkla et al. developed micelles that contain SPIONs and DOX and were used for cancer imaging and therapy [255]. Magnetoliposomes are the other nano-theranostics materials which are used for cancer therapy. Guo et al. designed a carboxymethyl dextran-coated magnetoliposome and used it for the delivery of DOX to human neuroblastoma SH-SY5Y cells. In this study they used low-frequency alternating magnetic field in order to increase the release of the drug without production of hyperthermia effect. In fact, SPIONs in this new system have played three roles: magnetic guide, MRI contrast agent, and affecting factor in drug release [256].

Proteins are another coating materials that are used in this field. Human serum albumin[26] has been used by Quan et al. as a cover for encapsulation of dopamine-coated iron oxide nanoparticles and DOX, simultaneously. They concluded that this new theranostic paradigm is a great platform for a range of lipophilic therapeutics [257].

The cavities of porous iron oxide nanoparticles are good area for loading anticancer drugs; Cheng et al. synthesized such a system for loading cisplatin and coupled it with Herceptin in order to be used for HER2 overexpressed breast cancer treatment [258].

Wang et al. prepared SPION-coated graphene oxide[27] and functionalized them with chitosan. This new nanoplatform with enhanced T2 contrast property was used for the co-delivery of DOX and plasmid DNA (p-DNA) to the cancer cells [259]. Yang et al. used SPIONs as a carrier for delivering siRNA. They coated silica-coated Fe_3O_4 nanoparticles $(Fe_3O_4@SiO_2)$ with a positive polymer (polyethylenimine[28]) and folic acid[29] as targeting agent. The electrostatic adsorption of siRNA onto $Fe_3O_4@SiO_2$/PEI-FA not only protected it from degradation by nucleases, but also made it to enter the specific cancer tissue more efficiently [260].

Thermoresponsive magnetic hydrogels like Fe_3O_4 encapsulated in the poly (NIPAAm) are also good candidates for cancer theranostics. Their intrinsic ability of shrinkage in response to the natural increase in the temperature of cancer tissues induced the drug release. As an example, in a research Jaiswal et al. used the thermal induction by MNPs for hydrogel's structural collapse [261].

Hyperthermia is the other therapeutic approach that has been used in the presence of SPIONs. According to this strategy, different types of SPION-based nanoparticle are introduced. Yallapu et al. synthesized a new system in which hyperthermia, chemotherapy, and MR imaging were conducted simultaneously. They used SPIONs decorated with multilayer β-cyclodextrin and pluronic polymer and curcumin as an anticancer drug [262].

---

[26]HSA.

[27]GO.

[28]PEI.

[29]FA.

SPIONs also could load photosensitizer agents for PDT; Reddy et al. utilized multifunctional polymeric nano-theranostics containing iron oxide and photofrin (as a photosensitizer agent) that are encapsulated in polyacrylamide and PEG, functionalized with F3 peptides for brain tumor-targeting [263].

Conjugation of two or more nanoparticles in one platform is another strategy to produce nano-theranostics agents that present new/better therapeutic effects with more sensitive diagnosis approaches. Yang et al. prepared a nanocomposite based on SPIONs and reduced graphene oxide[30] which was coated with PEG and used it as a nano-theranostics probe for in vivo photothermal therapy that was guided with MR imaging [264]. Another nano-theranostics system that is synthesized based on MNPs for photothermal treatment is PEGylated $Fe@Fe_3O_4$ which is introduced by Zhou et al. and induced apoptosis and necrosis in cancer cell in the presence of NIR laser irradiation [265]. Nanocomposite of upconversion nanoparticles and SPIONs has the potential to be used as multimodal imaging photothermal activator that uses NIR irradiation for luminescence imaging and therapy [266]. Au coating layer as photothermal absorber in any nanoplatform could induce photothermal therapeutic effect, $Fe_3O_4@hybrid@Au$ (introduced by Dong and his colleagues) is an example of this system that benefits from MR imaging property of Fe_3O_4 nanoparticles in combination with therapeutic property of Au [267].

Nanobubbles conjugated to the SPIONs were the next nano-theranostics platforms that used high-intensity focused US-triggered drug release and also US and MRI for image-guided therapy [268].

Huang et al. synthesized $\gamma Fe_2O_3@Au$ magnetic gold nanoflowers (MG NFs) as PTT nanotheraputic agents in which three different diagnostic approaches could be applied for monitoring the therapeutic process, photoacoustic[31] waves, MRI, and SERS [269].

1.3.2.5 SPIONs Based Nano-Theranostics for Inflammation, Neurodegenerative and Autoimmune Disease

Inflammation is the other field in which SPIONs could be used as nano-theranostics agents. In fact, SPIONs have been widely used as diagnostic material for stroke, atherosclerosis, angiography, and cardiovascular disease, but there exists limited researches that used these nanoparticles for simultaneous therapeutic and diagnostic applications of such diseases. In a recent research, Calle et al. used magnetoliposome for delivering omega-3 polyunsaturated fatty acid ethyl ester to the colonic inflammation which is attributed to glioma development and allowed MRI visualization of therapeutic process. Results showed significant decrease in the inflammatory effects and even reversing the development of glioma [270].

---

[30]rGO.
[31]PA.

Fu et al. applied SPION as a carrier for delivering anti-interleukin-1β mono-clonal antibody (anti-IL-1β mAb) to the epileptogenic tissues of brain. Anti-IL-1β mAb is an anti-inflammatory drug for brain inflammation which is synthesized against IL-1β derived from activated glial cells. They delivered the antibody to the targeted tissue through magnetic targeting, monitoring the inflammatory tissue through MRI, and suppress the inflammation simultaneously [271].

Since SPIONs could pass from blood–brain barrier (BBB), it can be applied for monitoring and delivering drugs to the unhealthy tissues in the central nervous system (CNS), among them is neurodegenerative disease. Moraes et al. used SPION-labeled mesenchymal stem cells for investigating their effects on decreasing the significances of Huntington's disease. Results showed that there is a significant decrease in the number of degenerating neurons at the target damaged tissue as well as an increase in the expression of fibroblast growth factor.[32] Moreover, the presence of iron oxide nanoparticles provided the feasibility of MR imaging of the striatum for at least 60 days after cell transplantation enabling cell tracking therapy for this nano-theranostics system [272].

Autoimmune diseases like type 1 diabetes appeared due to the activation of immune system of the body against its own cells, maybe because of an inflam-mation reaction which leads to the destruction of the cells of the affected tissue. Early detection and treating these diseases could eliminate their undesirable effects and restore the tissue functions. In this regard, theranostics nanoplatforms can play a dramatic role due to their simultaneous therapeutic and diagnostic properties. Wang et al. synthesized a dextran-coated iron oxide nanoparticles carrier and modified it with probes of siRNA which are active against human caspase-3 and assessed its effect on destruction of islet of the pancreas. In vivo MRI results demonstrated that the presence of siRNA prevent the apoptotic process of cells due to the decrease in the level of caspase-3 expression [273].

1.4 Challenges and Future Prospects

Nano-Theranostics phenomenon was emerged by employing nanomaterials for therapeutic and diagnostic applications as the same time. Among different types of nanomaterials, SPIONs could be widely used for nano-theranostics applications due to its particular properties such as superparamagnetism, ease of manufacturing, biodegradability, economic efficiency, remote controlling, self-diagnostic and therapeutic activity [274].

As a nano-theranostics agent which should be used inside the body, investigation on different properties of SPIONs and their effects on the body are critical steps that could be wrapped up through multiple safety and toxicological studies. Size, shape,

---

[32]FGF.

charge, surface properties, the route, and dose of administration are some of these considerable parameters.

The key point about bare SPIONs is their inherent tendency for aggregation which could limit their distribution in the circulatory system by the reticuloendothelial macrophages. Surface engineering of the nanoparticles with appropriate ligands, especially hydrophilic polymers, could not only prevent the aggregation process but also provides some other properties enhancing the theranostics application of these nanoparticles [275].

Another concern about the clinical applications of SPIONs is the adsorption of plasma proteins on the surface of the material, which is known as corona effect. The interaction between these proteins and SPIONs affects the pharmacological and biological properties of the nanoparticles, accelerating the plasmatic deletion of the SPIONs due to the enhancement in the attraction of immune cells. Till now, a wide variety of researches have been conducted on this issue to explain the best surface coating polymer with no corona effect [276, 277].

The obscure point about SPIONs is their dose-dependent cytotoxicity effect; in fact in some researches it was demonstrated that SPIONs at concentration above $100 \ \mu g \ ml^{-1}$ could induce cytotoxicity effect while other researches expressed that these nanoparticles have no toxicity effect on the viability of cells [278, 279]. Generation of ROS and oxidative stress, which could affect the performance of intracellular components and organelles, is the main reason of these researches for SPIONs toxicity feature. Indeed, lysosomal enzymes degrade the SPIONs content of endocytosis vesicle into Fe^{2+} ions. Based on the Fenton reaction, these ions could generate free hydroxyl radicals in reaction with hydrogen peroxide (Eqs. 1.1, 1.2), which can damage the cellular components.

$$Fe^{2+} + H_2O_2 + H^+ \rightarrow Fe^{3+} + HO^. + H_2O \tag{1.1}$$

$$Fe^{3+} + H_2O_2 \rightarrow Fe^{2+} + HOO^. + H^+ \tag{1.2}$$

Except dose, some other properties of SPIONs like hydrodynamic size, time of exposure, shape, and type of affected cells could also influence the toxicity level of SPIONs [280–282].

In general, more researches must be conducted and several other challenges must be overcome before introducing SPIONs as a trustful nano-theranostics agents for clinical applications. The ability to comply with the conditions of body and its immune system, delivering the therapeutic agent to the targeted site without leaving any side effect for other tissues, and imaging the disease tissue before and during the therapeutic process are critical features of nano-theranostics platforms. It is suggested that the next generation of SPION nano-theranostics agents are synthesis based on coupling multimodal imaging and multitherapeutic capabilities which are delivered to the targeted tissue through the use of active targeting agents in order to produce more sensitive device with high-performance therapeutic activity which could be used in the deepest parts of the body and also can overcome multidrug resistance of pathogenic disease [283].

References

1. Z. Dai, *Advances in Nanotheranostics I: Design and Fabrication of Theranosic Nanoparticles* (Springer, Berlin, 2015)
2. K.Y. Choi, G. Liu, S. Lee, X. Chen, Theranostic nanoplatforms for simultaneous cancer imaging and therapy: current approaches and future perspectives. Nanoscale **4**, 330–342 (2012)
3. Y. Zhou, X. Liang, Z. Dai, Porphyrin-loaded nanoparticles for cancer theranostics. Nanoscale **8**, 12394–12405 (2016)
4. Q. Chen, H. Ke, Z. Dai, Z. Liu, Nanoscale theranostics for physical stimulus-responsive cancer therapies. Biomaterials **73**, 214–230 (2015)
5. K. Greish, Enhanced permeability and retention (EPR) effect for anticancer nanomedicine drug targeting. Cancer Nanotechnol. Method. Protoc. **624**, 25–37 (2010)
6. X. Wu, Y. Gao, C.-M. Dong, Polymer/gold hybrid nanoparticles: from synthesis to cancer theranostic applications. RSC Advances **5**, 13787–13796 (2015)
7. D. Peer, J.M. Karp, S. Hong, O.C. Farokhzad, R. Margalit, R. Langer, Nanocarriers as an emerging platform for cancer therapy. Nat. Nanotechnol. **2**, 751–760 (2007)
8. S.K. Sahoo, V. Labhasetwar, Nanotech approaches to drug delivery and imaging. Drug Discovery Today **8**, 1112–1120 (2003)
9. J.T. Cole, N.B. Holland, Multifunctional nanoparticles for use in theranostic applications. Drug Deliv. Trans. Res. **5**, 295–309 (2015)
10. B. Semete, L. Booysen, Y. Lemmer, L. Kalombo, L. Katata, J. Verschoor, H.S. Swai, In vivo evaluation of the biodistribution and safety of PLGA nanoparticles as drug delivery systems. Nanomed. Nanotechnol. Biol. Med. **6**, 662–671 (2010)
11. H. Markides, M. Rotherham, A. El Haj, Biocompatibility and toxicity of magnetic nanoparticles in regenerative medicine. J. Nanomater. **2012**, 13 (2012)
12. M. Mahmoudi, A. Simchi, M. Imani, M.A. Shokrgozar, A.S. Milani, U.O. Häfeli, P. Stroeve, A new approach for the in vitro identification of the cytotoxicity of superparamagnetic iron oxide nanoparticles. Colloids Surf. B **75**, 300–309 (2010)
13. S. Parveen, R. Misra, S.K. Sahoo, Nanoparticles: a boon to drug delivery, therapeutics, diagnostics and imaging. Nanomed. Nanotechnol. Biol. Med. **8**, 147–166 (2012)
14. A. Kroll, M.H. Pillukat, D. Hahn, J. Schnekenburger, Current in vitro methods in nanoparticle risk assessment: limitations and challenges. Eur. J. Pharm. Biopharm. **72**, 370–377 (2009)
15. S.S. Kelkar, T.M. Reineke, Theranostics: combining imaging and therapy. Biocon. Chem. **22**, 1879–1903 (2011)
16. J. Wang, Y. Gao, Y. Hou, F. Zhao, F. Pu, X. Liu, Z. Wu, Y. Fan, Evaluation on cartilage morphology after intra-articular injection of titanium dioxide nanoparticles in rats. J. Nanomater. **2012**, 1–11 (2012)
17. S. Neethirajan, D.S. Jayas, Nanotechnology for the food and bioprocessing industries. Food Bioprocess Technol. **4**, 39–47 (2011)
18. Q. Huang, H. Yu, Q. Ru, Bioavailability and delivery of nutraceuticals using nanotechnology. J. Food Sci. **75**, R50–R57 (2010)
19. V. Sanna, N. Pala, M. Sechi, Targeted therapy using nanotechnology: focus on cancer. Int J. Nanomed. **9**, 467–483 (2014)
20. T.L. Doane, C. Burda, The unique role of nanoparticles in nanomedicine: imaging, drug delivery and therapy. Chem. Soc. Rev. **41**, 2885–2911 (2012)
21. B.Y. Kim, J.T. Rutka, W.C. Chan, Nanomedicine. N. Engl. J. Med. **363**, 2434–2443 (2010)
22. Y. Gao, J. Xie, H. Chen, S. Gu, R. Zhao, J. Shao, L. Jia, Nanotechnology-based intelligent drug design for cancer metastasis treatment. Biotechnol. Adv. **32**, 761–777 (2014)
23. M.J. Sailor, J.H. Park, Hybrid nanoparticles for detection and treatment of cancer. Adv. Mater. **24**, 3779–3802 (2012)

24. J.V. Jokerst, S.S. Gambhir, Molecular imaging with theranostic nanoparticles. Acc. Chem. Res. **44**, 1050–1060 (2011)

25. B. Fadeel, A.E. Garcia-Bennett, Better safe than sorry: understanding the toxicological properties of inorganic nanoparticles manufactured for biomedical applications. Adv. Drug Deliv. Rev. **62**, 362–374 (2010)

26. R. Singh, J.W. Lillard, Nanoparticle-based targeted drug delivery. Exp. Mol. Pathol. **86**, 215–223 (2009)

27. C.P. McCoy, C. Brady, J.F. Cowley, S.M. McGlinchey, N. McGoldrick, D.J. Kinnear, G.P. Andrews, D.S. Jones, Triggered drug delivery from biomaterials. Expert Opin. Drug Deliv. **7**, 605–616 (2010)

28. P. Rai, S. Mallidi, X. Zheng, R. Rahmanzadeh, Y. Mir, S. Elrington, A. Khurshid, T. Hasan, Development and applications of photo-triggered theranostic agents. Adv. Drug Deliv. Rev. **62**, 1094–1124 (2010)

29. K.H. Martin, P.A. Dayton, Current status and prospects for microbubbles in ultrasound theranostics. Wiley Interdiscip. Rev. Nanomed. Nanobiotechnol. **5**, 329–345 (2013)

30. R.R. Ragheb, D. Kim, A. Bandyopadhyay, H. Chahboune, B. Bulutoglu, H. Ezaldein, J.M. Criscione, T.M. Fahmy, Induced clustered nanoconfinement of superparamagnetic iron oxide in biodegradable nanoparticles enhances transverse relaxivity for targeted theranostics. Magn. Reson. Med. **70**, 1748–1760 (2013)

31. D. Maity, S.-G. Choo, J. Yi, J. Ding, J.M. Xue, Synthesis of magnetite nanoparticles via a solvent-free thermal decomposition route. J. Magn. Magn. Mater. **321**, 1256–1259 (2009)

32. S. Shen, S. Wang, R. Zheng, X. Zhu, X. Jiang, D. Fu, W. Yang, Magnetic nanoparticle clusters for photothermal therapy with near-infrared irradiation. Biomaterials **39**, 67–74 (2015)

33. J. Wan, W. Cai, X. Meng, E. Liu, Monodisperse water-soluble magnetite nanoparticles prepared by polyol process for high-performance magnetic resonance imaging. Chem. Commun. **47**, 5004–5006 (2007)

34. D. Ho, X. Sun, S. Sun, Monodisperse magnetic nanoparticles for theranostic applications. Acc. Chem. Res. **44**, 875–882 (2011)

35. A.J. Cole, V.C. Yang, A.E. David, Cancer theranostics: the rise of targeted magnetic nanoparticles. Trends Biotechnol. **29**, 323–332 (2011)

36. A.H. Lu, E.E.L. Salabas, F. Schüth, Magnetic nanoparticles: synthesis, protection, functionalization, and application. Angew. Chem. Int. Ed. **46**, 1222–1244 (2007)

37. M. Faraji, Y. Yamini, M. Rezaee, Magnetic nanoparticles: synthesis, stabilization, functionalization, characterization, and applications. J. Iran. Chem. Soc. **7**, 1–37 (2010)

38. C. Okoli, Development of protein-functionalized magnetic iron oxide nanoparticles: potential application in water treatment, Doctoral thesis, 2012

39. D. Caruntu, G. Caruntu, C.J. O'Connor, Magnetic properties of variable-sized Fe_3O_4 nanoparticles synthesized from non-aqueous homogeneous solutions of polyols. J. Phys. D Appl. Phys. **40**, 5801–5810 (2007)

40. A.K. Gupta, M. Gupta, Synthesis and surface engineering of iron oxide nanoparticles for biomedical applications. Biomaterials **26**, 3995–4021 (2005)

41. S. Sun, H. Zeng, Size-controlled synthesis of magnetite nanoparticles. J. Am. Chem. Soc. **124**, 8204–8205 (2002)

42. R. Hao, R. Xing, Z. Xu, Y. Hou, S. Gao, S. Sun, Synthesis, functionalization, and biomedical applications of multifunctional magnetic nanoparticles. Adv. Mater. **22**, 2729–2742 (2010)

43. P. Tartaj, M. del Puerto Morales, S. Veintemillas-Verdaguer, T. González-Carreño, C. J. Serna, The preparation of magnetic nanoparticles for applications in biomedicine. J. Phys. D Appl. Phys. **36**, R182–R198 (2003)

44. J. Sun, S. Zhou, P. Hou, Y. Yang, J. Weng, X. Li, M. Li, Synthesis and characterization of biocompatible Fe_3O_4 nanoparticles. J. Biomed. Mater. Res., Part A **80**, 333–341 (2007)

45. Z. Liu, Y. Liu, K. Yao, Z. Ding, J. Tao, X. Wang, Synthesis and magnetic properties of Fe_3O_4 nanoparticles. J. Mater. Synth. Process. **10**, 83–87 (2002)

46. E. Bertolucci, A.M.R. Galletti, C. Antonetti, F. Piccinelli, M. Marracci, B. Tellini, C. Visone, Chemical and magnetic properties characterization of magnetic nanoparticles, in *Instrumentation and Measurement Technology Conference (I2MTC), IEEE International* (2015), pp. 1492–1496

47. V. Dolgovskiy, V. Lebedev, S. Colombo, A. Weis, B. Michen, L. Ackermann-Hirschi, A. Petri-Fink, A quantitative study of particle size effects in the magnetorelaxometry of magnetic nanoparticles using atomic magnetometry. J. Magn. Magn. Mater. **379**, 137–150 (2015)

48. K.C.-F. Leung, S. Xuan, Y.J. Wang, From micro to nano magnetic spheres: size-controllable synthesis. Multilayer Coat. Biomed. Appl. **13**, 15 (2016)

49. P.I. Soares, F. Lochte, C. Echeverria, L.C. Pereira, J.T. Coutinho, I.M. Ferreira, C.M. Novo, Thermal and magnetic properties of iron oxide colloids: influence of surfactants. Nanotechnology **26**, 425704 (2015)

50. K.L. Aillon, Y. Xie, N. El-Gendy, C.J. Berkland, M.L. Forrest, Effects of nanomaterial physicochemical properties on in vivo toxicity. Adv. Drug Deliv. Rev. **61**, 457–466 (2009)

51. C.C. Berry, S. Wells, S. Charles, A.S. Curtis, Dextran and albumin derivatised iron oxide nanoparticles: influence on fibroblasts in vitro. Biomaterials **24**, 4551–4557 (2003)

52. A. Verma, F. Stellacci, Effect of surface properties on nanoparticle–cell interactions. Small **6**, 12–21 (2010)

53. J. Huang, L. Bu, J. Xie, K. Chen, Z. Cheng, X. Li, X. Chen, Effects of nanoparticle size on cellular uptake and liver MRI with polyvinylpyrrolidone-coated iron oxide nanoparticles. ACS Nano **4**, 7151–7160 (2010)

54. D. Stanicki, L. Vander Elst, R.N. Muller, S. Laurent, Synthesis and processing of magnetic nanoparticles. Curr. Opin. Chem. Eng. **8**, 7–14 (2015)

55. C. Corot, P. Robert, J.-M. Idée, M. Port, Recent advances in iron oxide nanocrystal technology for medical imaging. Adv. Drug Deliv. Rev. **58**, 1471–1504 (2006)

56. L.H. Reddy, J.L. Arias, J. Nicolas, P. Couvreur, Magnetic nanoparticles: design and characterization, toxicity and biocompatibility, pharmaceutical and biomedical applications. Chem. Rev. **112**, 5818–5878 (2012)

57. X. Li, W. Liu, L. Sun, K.E. Aifantis, B. Yu, Y. Fan, Q. Feng, F. Cui, F. Watari, Effects of physicochemical properties of nanomaterials on their toxicity. J. Biomed. Mater. Res., Part A **103**, 2499–2507 (2015)

58. K. Xiao, Y. Li, J. Luo, J.S. Lee, W. Xiao, A.M. Gonik, R.G. Agarwal, K.S. Lam, The effect of surface charge on in vivo biodistribution of PEG-oligocholic acid based micellar nanoparticles. Biomaterials **32**, 3435–3446 (2011)

59. M. Kim, J. Jung, J. Lee, K. Na, S. Park, J. Hyun, Amphiphilic comblike polymers enhance the colloidal stability of Fe_3O_4 nanoparticles. Colloids Surf., B **76**, 236–240 (2010)

60. M. Szekeres, I.Y. Tóth, E. Illés, A. Hajdú, I. Zupkó, K. Farkas, G. Oszlánczi, L. Tiszlavicz, E. Tombácz, Chemical and colloidal stability of carboxylated core-shell magnetite nanoparticles designed for biomedical applications. Int. J. Mol. Sci. **14**, 14550–14574 (2013)

61. S. Ghosh, W. Jiang, J.D. McClements, B. Xing, Colloidal stability of magnetic iron oxide nanoparticles: influence of natural organic matter and synthetic polyelectrolytes. Langmuir **27**, 8036–8043 (2011)

62. D. Singh, J.M. McMillan, X.-M. Liu, H.M. Vishwasrao, A.V. Kabanov, M. Sokolsky-Papkov, H.E. Gendelman, Formulation design facilitates magnetic nanoparticle delivery to diseased cells and tissues. Nanomedicine **9**, 469–485 (2014)

63. S. Laurent, D. Forge, M. Port, A. Roch, C. Robic, L. Van der Elst, R.N. Muller, Magnetic iron oxide nanoparticles: synthesis, stabilization, vectorization, physicochemical characterizations, and biological applications. Chem. Rev. **108**, 2064–2110 (2008)

64. S. Mornet, J. Portier, E. Duguet, A method for synthesis and functionalization of ultrasmall superparamagnetic covalent carriers based on maghemite and dextran. J. Magn. Magn. Mater. **293**, 127–134 (2005)

65. L. LaConte, N. Nitin, G. Bao, Magnetic nanoparticle probes. Mater. Today **8**, 32–38 (2005)

66. A.A. Ismail, Synthesis and characterization of $Y_2O_3/Fe_2O_3/TiO_2$ nanoparticles by sol–gel method. Appl. Catal. B **58**, 115–121 (2005)
67. Z. Dai, F. Meiser, H. Möhwald, Nanoengineering of iron oxide and iron oxide/silica hollow spheres by sequential layering combined with a sol–gel process. J. Colloid Interface Sci. **288**, 298–300 (2005)
68. A.S. Teja, P.-Y. Koh, Synthesis, properties, and applications of magnetic iron oxide nanoparticles. Prog. Cryst. Growth Charact. Mater. **55**, 22–45 (2009)
69. A. Roca, M. Morales, K. O'Grady, C. Serna, Structural and magnetic properties of uniform magnetite nanoparticles prepared by high temperature decomposition of organic precursors. Nanotechnology **17**, 2783 (2006)
70. Z. Xu, C. Shen, Y. Hou, H. Gao, S. Sun, Oleylamine as both reducing agent and stabilizer in a facile synthesis of magnetite nanoparticles. Chem. Mater. **21**, 1778–1780 (2009)
71. P. Tartaj, M.P. Morales, S. Veintemillas-Verdaguer, T. Gonzalez-Carreño, C.J. Serna, Synthesis, properties and biomedical applications of magnetic nanoparticles. Handbook Magn. Mater. **16**, 403–482 (2006)
72. W. Cai, J. Wan, Facile synthesis of superparamagnetic magnetite nanoparticles in liquid polyols. J. Colloid Interface Sci. **305**, 366–370 (2007)
73. J. Merikhi, H.-O. Jungk, C. Feldmann, Sub-micrometer $CoAl_2O_4$ pigment particles—synthesis and preparation of coatings. J. Mater. Chem. **10**, 1311–1314 (2000)
74. S.-J. Park, S. Kim, S. Lee, Z.G. Khim, K. Char, T. Hyeon, Synthesis and magnetic studies of uniform iron nanorods and nanospheres. J. Am. Chem. Soc. **122**, 8581–8582 (2000)
75. R.A. Mukh-Qasem, A. Gedanken, Sonochemical synthesis of stable hydrosol of Fe_3O_4 nanoparticles. J. Colloid Interface Sci. **284**, 489–494 (2005)
76. E.H. Kim, H.S. Lee, B.K. Kwak, B.-K. Kim, Synthesis of ferrofluid with magnetic nanoparticles by sonochemical method for MRI contrast agent. J. Magn. Magn. Mater. **289**, 328–330 (2005)
77. W. Wu, Q. He, C. Jiang, Magnetic iron oxide nanoparticles: synthesis and surface functionalization strategies. Nanoscale Res. Lett. **3**, 397–415 (2008)
78. Y.-H. Zheng, Y. Cheng, F. Bao, Y.-S. Wang, Synthesis and magnetic properties of Fe_3O_4 nanoparticles. Mater. Res. Bull. **41**, 525–529 (2006)
79. X. Wang, J. Zhuang, Q. Peng, Y. Li, A general strategy for nanocrystal synthesis. Nature **437**, 121–124 (2005)
80. H. Cai, X. An, J. Cui, J. Li, S. Wen, K. Li, M. Shen, L. Zheng, G. Zhang, X. Shi, Facile hydrothermal synthesis and surface functionalization of polyethyleneimine-coated iron oxide nanoparticles for biomedical applications. ACS Appl. Mater. Interfaces **5**, 1722–1731 (2013)
81. B.K. Paul, S.P. Moulik, Uses and applications of microemulsions. Curr. Sci. Bangalore **80**, 990–1001 (2001)
82. M. Darbandi, F. Stromberg, J. Landers, N. Reckers, B. Sanyal, W. Keune, H. Wende, Nanoscale size effect on surface spin canting in iron oxide nanoparticles synthesized by the microemulsion method. J. Phys. D Appl. Phys. **45**, 195001 (2012)
83. S. Ghorbanzadeh-Mashkani, P. Tajer-Mohammad-Ghazvini, A. Nozad-Golikand, R. Kasra-Kermanshahi, M.-R. Davarpanah, Synthesis of sterile and pyrogen free biogenic magnetic nanoparticles: biotechnological potential of magnetotactic bacteria for production of nanomaterials, in *Proceedings of World Academy of Science, Engineering and Technology, World Academy of Science, Engineering and Technology (WASET)*, vol. 74 (2013), pp. 194–198
84. C. Prasad, K. Sreenivasulu, S. Gangadhara, P. Venkateswarlu, A facile green synthesis of spherical Fe_3O_4 magnetic nanoparticles and their effect on degradation of methylene blue in aqueous solution. J. Mol. Liq. **221**, 993–998 (2016)
85. M. Mahdavi, F. Namvar, M.B. Ahmad, R. Mohamad, Green biosynthesis and characterization of magnetic iron oxide (Fe_3O_4) nanoparticles using seaweed (Sargassum muticum) aqueous extract. Molecules **18**, 5954–5964 (2013)
86. J. Dobson, Magnetic nanoparticles for drug delivery. Drug Dev. Res. **67**, 55–60 (2006)

87. A. Ito, M. Kamihira, Tissue engineering using magnetite nanoparticles. Progr. Mol. Biol. Trans. Sci. **104**, 355–395 (2010)
88. Š. Kubinová, E. Syková, Nanotechnologies in regenerative medicine. Minim. Invasive Ther. Allied Technol. **19**, 144–156 (2010)
89. N. Bock, A. Riminucci, C. Dionigi, A. Russo, A. Tampieri, E. Landi, V.A. Goranov, M. Marcacci, V. Dediu, A novel route in bone tissue engineering: magnetic biomimetic scaffolds. Acta Biomater. **6**, 786–796 (2010)
90. M. Ishii, R. Shibata, Y. Numaguchi, T. Kito, H. Suzuki, K. Shimizu, A. Ito, H. Honda, T. Murohara, Enhanced angiogenesis by transplantation of mesenchymal stem cell sheet created by a novel magnetic tissue engineering method. Arterioscler. Thromb. Vasc. Biol. **31**, 2210–2215 (2011)
91. M. Mahmoudi, M. Zhao, Y. Matsuura, S. Laurent, P.C. Yang, D. Bernstein, P. Ruiz-Lozano, V. Serpooshan, Infection-resistant MRI-visible scaffolds for tissue engineering applications. BioImpacts: BI **6**, 111–115 (2016)
92. V. Kandi, S. Kandi, Antimicrobial properties of nanomolecules: potential candidates as antibiotics in the era of multi-drug resistance. Epidemiol. Health **37**, e2015020 (2015)
93. E.N. Taylor, K.M. Kummer, N.G. Durmus, K. Leuba, K.M. Tarquinio, T.J. Webster, Superparamagnetic Iron Oxide Nanoparticles (SPION) for the treatment of antibiotic-resistant biofilms. Small **8**, 3016–3027 (2012)
94. T. Sasaki, N. Iwasaki, K. Kohno, M. Kishimoto, T. Majima, S.I. Nishimura, A. Minami, Magnetic nanoparticles for improving cell invasion in tissue engineering. J. Biomed. Mater. Res., Part A **86**, 969–978 (2008)
95. A. Ito, H. Akiyama, Y. Kawabe, M. Kamihira, Magnetic force-based cell patterning using Arg-Gly-Asp (RGD) peptide-conjugated magnetite cationic liposomes. J. Biosci. Bioeng. **104**, 288–293 (2007)
96. A. Ito, Y. Takizawa, H. Honda, K.-I. Hata, H. Kagami, M. Ueda, T. Kobayashi, Tissue engineering using magnetite nanoparticles and magnetic force: heterotypic layers of cocultured hepatocytes and endothelial cells. Tissue Eng. **10**, 833–840 (2004)
97. E.A. Lee, H. Yim, J. Heo, H. Kim, G. Jung, N.S. Hwang, Application of magnetic nanoparticle for controlled tissue assembly and tissue engineering. Arch. Pharmacal Res. **37**, 120–128 (2014)
98. Y. Gao, J. Lim, S.-H. Teoh, C. Xu, Emerging translational research on magnetic nanoparticles for regenerative medicine. Chem. Soc. Rev. **44**, 6306–6329 (2015)
99. G.R. Souza, J.R. Molina, R.M. Raphael, M.G. Ozawa, D.J. Stark, C.S. Levin, L.F. Bronk, J. S. Ananta, J. Mandelin, M.-M. Georgescu, Three-dimensional tissue culture based on magnetic cell levitation. Nat. Nanotechnol. **5**, 291–296 (2010)
100. L.J. Santos, R.L. Reis, M.E. Gomes, Harnessing magnetic-mechano actuation in regenerative medicine and tissue engineering. Trends Biotechnol. **33**, 471–479 (2015)
101. L. Borlido, A. Azevedo, A. Roque, M. Aires-Barros, Magnetic separations in biotechnology. Biotechnol. Adv. **31**, 1374–1385 (2013)
102. I. Safarik, M. Safarikova, Magnetic techniques for the isolation and purification of proteins and peptides. BioMagn. Res. Technol. **2**, 1–17 (2004)
103. P.A. Liberti, C.G. Rao, L.W. Terstappen, Optimization of ferrofluids and protocols for the enrichment of breast tumor cells in blood. J. Magn. Magn. Mater. **225**, 301–307 (2001)
104. Q.A. Pankhurst, J. Connolly, S.K. Jones, J. Dobson, Applications of magnetic nanoparticles in biomedicine. J. Phys. D Appl. Phys. **36**, R167 (2003)
105. A.H. Latham, M.E. Williams, Controlling transport and chemical functionality of magnetic nanoparticles. Acc. Chem. Res. **41**, 411–420 (2008)
106. K. Hola, Z. Markova, G. Zoppellaro, J. Tucek, R. Zboril, Tailored functionalization of iron oxide nanoparticles for MRI, drug delivery, magnetic separation and immobilization of biosubstances. Biotechnol. Adv. **33**, 1162–1176 (2015)

107. J. He, M. Huang, D. Wang, Z. Zhang, G. Li, Magnetic separation techniques in sample preparation for biological analysis: a review. J. Pharm. Biomed. Anal. **101**, 84–101 (2014)
108. F. Wang, Y. Hu, C. Guo, W. Huang, C.-Z. Liu, Enhanced phenol degradation in coking wastewater by immobilized laccase on magnetic mesoporous silica nanoparticles in a magnetically stabilized fluidized bed. Bioresour. Technol. **110**, 120–124 (2012)
109. M. Uyttendaele, I. Van Hoorde, J. Debevere, The use of immuno-magnetic separation (IMS) as a tool in a sample preparation method for direct detection of L. monocytogenes in cheese. Int. J. Food Microbiol. **54**, 205–212 (2000)
110. J.R. Wisniewski, A. Zougman, N. Nagaraj, M. Mann, Universal sample preparation method for proteome analysis. Nat. Methods **6**, 359–362 (2009)
111. M. Colombo, S. Carregal-Romero, M.F. Casula, L. Gutierrez, M.P. Morales, I.B. Boehm, J.T. Heverhagen, D. Prosperi, W.J. Parak, Biological applications of magnetic nanoparticles. Chem. Soc. Rev. **41**, 4306–4334 (2012)
112. J.-C. Leroux, Injectable nanocarriers for biodetoxification. Nat. Nanotechnol. **2**, 679–684 (2007)
113. M.D. Kaminski, A.J. Rosengart, Detoxification of blood using injectable magnetic nanospheres: a conceptual technology description. J. Magn. Magn. Mater. **293**, 398–403 (2005)
114. M. Rahman, A.A. Saei, H. Amiri, M. Mahmoudi, Biomedical applications of superparamagnetic nanoparticles in molecular scale. Curr. Org. Chem. **19**, 982–990 (2015)
115. L. Wang, Z. Yang, J. Gao, K. Xu, H. Gu, B. Zhang, X. Zhang, B. Xu, A biocompatible method of decorporation: bisphosphonate-modified magnetite nanoparticles to remove uranyl ions from blood. J. Am. Chem. Soc. **128**, 13358–13359 (2006)
116. J.-J. Lee, K.J. Jeong, M. Hashimoto, A.H. Kwon, A. Rwei, S.A. Shankarappa, J.H. Tsui, D.S. Kohane, Synthetic ligand-coated magnetic nanoparticles for microfluidic bacterial separation from blood. Nano Lett. **14**, 1–5 (2013)
117. H. Lee, T.J. Yoon, R. Weissleder, Ultrasensitive detection of bacteria using core-shell nanoparticles and an NMR-filter system. Angew. Chem. Int. Ed. **48**, 5657–5660 (2009)
118. K. El-Boubbou, C. Gruden, X. Huang, Magnetic glyco-nanoparticles: a unique tool for rapid pathogen detection, decontamination, and strain differentiation. J. Am. Chem. Soc. **129**, 13392–13393 (2007)
119. S. Ryan, A.J. Kell, H. van Faassen, L.-L. Tay, B. Simard, R. MacKenzie, M. Gilbert, J. Tanha, Single-domain antibody-nanoparticles: promising architectures for increased Staphylococcus aureus detection specificity and sensitivity. Biocon. Chem. **20**, 1966–1974 (2009)
120. C. Kaittanis, S.A. Naser, J.M. Perez, One-step, nanoparticle-mediated bacterial detection with magnetic relaxation. Nano Lett. **7**, 380–383 (2007)
121. S. Pal, E.C. Alocilja, Electrically active polyaniline coated magnetic (EAPM) nanoparticle as novel transducer in biosensor for detection of Bacillus anthracis spores in food samples. Biosens. Bioelectron. **24**, 1437–1444 (2009)
122. J. Gao, H. Gu, B. Xu, Multifunctional magnetic nanoparticles: design, synthesis, and biomedical applications. Acc. Chem. Res. **42**, 1097–1107 (2009)
123. H. Gu, K. Xu, C. Xu, B. Xu, Biofunctional magnetic nanoparticles for protein separation and pathogen detection. Chem. Commun. **9**, 941–949 (2006)
124. Q. Liu, J. Shi, M. Cheng, G. Li, D. Cao, G. Jiang, Preparation of graphene-encapsulated magnetic microspheres for protein/peptide enrichment and MALDI-TOF MS analysis. Chem. Commun. **48**, 1874–1876 (2012)
125. H. Chen, D. Qi, C. Deng, P. Yang, X. Zhang, Preparation of C60-functionalized magnetic silica microspheres for the enrichment of low-concentration peptides and proteins for MALDI-TOF MS analysis. Proteomics **9**, 380–387 (2009)
126. J.S. Kim, C.A. Valencia, R. Liu, W. Lin, Highly-efficient purification of native polyhistidine-tagged proteins by multivalent NTA-modified magnetic nanoparticles. Biocon. Chem. **18**, 333–341 (2007)

127. S. Mazzucchelli, M. Colombo, C. De Palma, A. Salvade, P. Verderio, M.D. Coghi, E. Clementi, P. Tortora, F. Corsi, D. Prosperi, Single-domain protein A-engineered magnetic nanoparticles: toward a universal strategy to site-specific labeling of antibodies for targeted detection of tumor cells. ACS Nano 4, 5693–5702 (2010)

128. H. Cai, X. Gu, M.S. Scanlan, C.R. Lively, Development of a quantitative PCR assay for residual mouse DNA and comparison of four sample purification methods for DNA isolation. J. Pharm. Biomed. Anal. 55, 71–77 (2011)

129. D. Leung, S.O. Kang, E.V. Anslyn, Rapid determination of enantiomeric excess: a focus on optical approaches. Chem. Soc. Rev. 41, 448–479 (2012)

130. J.W. Hong, V. Studer, G. Hang, W.F. Anderson, S.R. Quake, A nanoliter-scale nucleic acid processor with parallel architecture. Nat. Biotechnol. 22, 435–439 (2004)

131. A. Soozanipour, A. Taheri-Kafrani, A.L. Isfahani, Covalent attachment of xylanase on functionalized magnetic nanoparticles and determination of its activity and stability. Chem. Eng. J. 270, 235–243 (2015)

132. K. Khoshnevisan, A.-K. Bordbar, D. Zare, D. Davoodi, M. Noruzi, M. Barkhi, M. Tabatabaei, Immobilization of cellulase enzyme on superparamagnetic nanoparticles and determination of its activity and stability. Chem. Eng. J. 171, 669–673 (2011)

133. M. Pečová, M. Šebela, Z. Markova, K. Polakova, J. Čuda, K. Šafářová, R. Zbořil, Thermostable trypsin conjugates immobilized to biogenic magnetite show a high operational stability and remarkable reusability for protein digestion. Nanotechnology 24, 125102 (2013)

134. C.-C. Yu, Y.-Y. Kuo, C.-F. Liang, W.-T. Chien, H.-T. Wu, T.-C. Chang, F.-D. Jan, C.-C. Lin, Site-specific immobilization of enzymes on magnetic nanoparticles and their use in organic synthesis. Biocon. Chem. 23, 714–724 (2012)

135. S. Metz, G. Bonaterra, M. Rudelius, M. Settles, E.J. Rummeny, H.E. Daldrup-Link, Capacity of human monocytes to phagocytose approved iron oxide MR contrast agents in vitro. Eur. Radiol. 14, 1851–1858 (2004)

136. J.W. Bulte, Magnetic nanoparticles as markers for cellular MR imaging. J. Magn. Magn. Mater. 289, 423–427 (2005)

137. C. Zhang, T. Liu, J. Gao, Y. Su, C. Shi, Recent development and application of magnetic nanoparticles for cell labeling and imaging. Mini Rev. Med. Chem. 10, 194–203 (2010)

138. A.S. Arbab, G.T. Yocum, H. Kalish, E.K. Jordan, S.A. Anderson, A.Y. Khakoo, E.J. Read, J.A. Frank, Efficient magnetic cell labeling with protamine sulfate complexed to ferumoxides for cellular MRI. Blood 104, 1217–1223 (2004)

139. J.W. Bulte, T. Douglas, B. Witwer, S.-C. Zhang, E. Strable, B.K. Lewis, H. Zywicke, B. Miller, P. van Gelderen, B.M. Moskowitz, Magnetodendrimers allow endosomal magnetic labeling and in vivo tracking of stem cells. Nat. Biotechnol. 19, 1141–1147 (2001)

140. C.C. Berry, Progress in functionalization of magnetic nanoparticles for applications in biomedicine. J. Phys. D Appl. Phys. 42, 224003 (2009)

141. J.K. Herr, J.E. Smith, C.D. Medley, D. Shangguan, W. Tan, Aptamer-conjugated nanoparticles for selective collection and detection of cancer cells. Anal. Chem. 78, 2918–2924 (2006)

142. J.E. Jaetao, K.S. Butler, N.L. Adolphi, D.M. Lovato, H.C. Bryant, I. Rabinowitz, S.S. Winter, T.E. Tessier, H.J. Hathaway, C. Bergemann, Enhanced leukemia cell detection using a novel magnetic needle and nanoparticles. Cancer Res. 69, 8310–8316 (2009)

143. T. Kekarainen, S. Mannelin, J. Laine, T. Jaatinen, Optimization of immunomagnetic separation for cord blood-derived hematopoietic stem cells. BMC Cell Biol. 7, 1–10 (2006)

144. K. Pantel, C. Alix-Panabières, S. Riethdorf, Cancer micrometastases. Nat. Rev. Clin. Oncol. 6, 339–351 (2009)

145. V.I. Shubayev, T.R. Pisanic, S. Jin, Magnetic nanoparticles for theragnostics. Adv. Drug Deliv. Rev. 61, 467–477 (2009)

146. X. Chen, S.T. Wong, Cancer theranostics: An introduction. Cancer Theranostics, Chap. 1, 3–8 (2014)

147. B.T. Luk, L. Zhang, Current advances in polymer-based nanotheranostics for cancer treatment and diagnosis. ACS Appl. Mater. Interfaces **6**, 21859–21873 (2014)
148. M. Zheng, S. Liu, J. Li, D. Qu, H. Zhao, X. Guan, X. Hu, Z. Xie, X. Jing, Z. Sun, Integrating oxaliplatin with highly luminescent carbon dots: an unprecedented theranostic agent for personalized medicine. Adv. Mater. **26**, 3554–3560 (2014)
149. S.D. Jo, S.H. Ku, Y.-Y. Won, S.H. Kim, I.C. Kwon, Targeted nanotheranostics for future personalized medicine: recent progress in cancer therapy. Theranostics **6**, 1362–1377 (2016)
150. J. Xie, S. Lee, X. Chen, Nanoparticle-based theranostic agents. Adv. Drug Deliv. Rev. **62**, 1064–1079 (2010)
151. L.Y. Rizzo, B. Theek, G. Storm, F. Kiessling, T. Lammers, Recent progress in nanomedicine: therapeutic, diagnostic and theranostic applications. Curr. Opin. Biotechnol. **24**, 1159–1166 (2013)
152. T. Lammers, F. Kiessling, W.E. Hennink, G. Storm, Nanotheranostics and image-guided drug delivery: current concepts and future directions. Mol. Pharm. **7**, 1899–1912 (2010)
153. A. Radomska, J. Leszczyszyn, M.W. Radomski, The nanopharmacology and nanotoxicology of nanomaterials: new opportunities and challenges. Adv. Clin. Exp. Med. Off. Organ Wroclaw Med. Univ. **25**, 151 (2016)
154. S.M. Janib, A.S. Moses, J.A. MacKay, Imaging and drug delivery using theranostic nanoparticles. Adv. Drug Deliv. Rev. **62**, 1052–1063 (2010)
155. B.T. Luk, R.H. Fang, L. Zhang, Lipid-and polymer-based nanostructures for cancer theranostics. Theranostics **2**, 1117–1126 (2012)
156. M.S. Muthu, D.T. Leong, L. Mei, S.-S. Feng, Nanotheranostics-application and further development of nanomedicine strategies for advanced theranostics. Theranostics **4**, 660–677 (2014)
157. T.H. Kim, S. Lee, X. Chen, Nanotheranostics for personalized medicine. Expert Rev. Mol. Diagn. **13**, 257–269 (2013)
158. Z.-P. Liang, P.C. Lauterbur, *Principles of Magnetic Resonance Imaging: A Signal Processing Perspective* (The Institute of Electrical and Electronics Engineers Press, 2000)
159. J. Hsieh, *Computed Tomography: Principles, Design, Artifacts, and Recent Advances* (SPIE Bellingham, WA, 2009)
160. M.E. Phelps, Positron emission tomography provides molecular imaging of biological processes. Proc. Natl. Acad. Sci. **97**, 9226–9233 (2000)
161. T.A. Holly, B.G. Abbott, M. Al-Mallah, D.A. Calnon, M.C. Cohen, F.P. DiFilippo, E.P. Ficaro, M.R. Freeman, R.C. Hendel, D. Jain, Single photon-emission computed tomography. J. Nucl. Cardiol. **17**, 941–973 (2010)
162. C.R. Hill, J.C. Bamber, G. ter Haar, *Physical Principles of Medical Ultrasonics* (Wiley Online Library, 2004)
163. M. Gu, *Advanced Optical Imaging Theory* (Springer Science & Business Media, 2000)
164. G. Bao, S. Mitragotri, S. Tong, Multifunctional nanoparticles for drug delivery and molecular imaging. Annu. Rev. Biomed. Eng. **15**, 253–282 (2013)
165. Y. Bao, T. Wen, A.C.S. Samia, A. Khandhar, K.M. Krishnan, Magnetic nanoparticles: material engineering and emerging applications in lithography and biomedicine. J. Mater. Sci. **51**, 513–553 (2016)
166. N.A. Frey, S. Peng, K. Cheng, S. Sun, Magnetic nanoparticles: synthesis, functionalization, and applications in bioimaging and magnetic energy storage. Chem. Soc. Rev. **38**, 2532–2542 (2009)
167. T. Neuberger, B. Schöpf, H. Hofmann, M. Hofmann, B. Von Rechenberg, Superparamagnetic nanoparticles for biomedical applications: possibilities and limitations of a new drug delivery system. J. Magn. Magn. Mater. **293**, 483–496 (2005)
168. M.F. Kircher, J.K. Willmann, Molecular body imaging: MR imaging, CT, and US. Part I. Principles. Radiology **263**, 633–643 (2012)
169. J.K. Willmann, N. van Bruggen, L.M. Dinkelborg, S.S. Gambhir, Molecular imaging in drug development. Nat. Rev. Drug Discov. **7**, 591–607 (2008)

170. N. Lee, T. Hyeon, Designed synthesis of uniformly sized iron oxide nanoparticles for efficient magnetic resonance imaging contrast agents. Chem. Soc. Rev. **41**, 2575–2589 (2012)

171. N. Lee, D. Yoo, D. Ling, M.H. Cho, T. Hyeon, J. Cheon, Iron oxide based nanoparticles for multimodal imaging and magnetoresponsive therapy. Chem. Rev. **115**, 10637–10689 (2015)

172. Z.R. Stephen, F.M. Kievit, M. Zhang, Magnetite nanoparticles for medical MR imaging. Mater. Today **14**, 330–338 (2011)

173. P. Gatehouse, G. Bydder, Magnetic resonance imaging of short T2 components in tissue. Clin. Radiol. **58**, 1–19 (2003)

174. M.M. Britton, Magnetic resonance imaging of chemistry. Chem. Soc. Rev. **39**, 4036–4043 (2010)

175. P. Caravan, C.T. Farrar, L. Frullano, R. Uppal, Influence of molecular parameters and increasing magnetic field strength on relaxivity of gadolinium-and manganese-based T1 contrast agents. Contrast Media Mol. Imaging **4**, 89–100 (2009)

176. Y.W. Jun, J.H. Lee, J. Cheon, Chemical design of nanoparticle probes for high-performance magnetic resonance imaging. Angewandte Chemie International Edition, **47**, 5122–5135 (2008)

177. M.K. Uchiyama, S.H. Toma, S.F. de Paula Rodrigues, A.L.B. Shimada, R.A. Loiola, H.J.C. Rodríguez, P.V. Oliveira, M.S. Luz, S.R. Rabbani, H.E. Toma, Ultrasmall cationic superparamagnetic iron oxide nanoparticles as nontoxic and efficient MRI contrast agent and magnetic-targeting tool. Int. J. Nanomed. **10**, 4731–4746 (2015)

178. P. Reimer, T. Balzer, Ferucarbotran (Resovist): a new clinically approved RES-specific contrast agent for contrast-enhanced MRI of the liver: properties, clinical development, and applications. Eur. Radiol. **13**, 1266–1276 (2003)

179. J.R. McCarthy, R. Weissleder, Multifunctional magnetic nanoparticles for targeted imaging and therapy. Adv. Drug Deliv. Rev. **60**, 1241–1251 (2008)

180. M. Longmire, P.L. Choyke, H. Kobayashi, *Clearance Properties of Nano-Sized Particles and Molecules as Imaging Agents: Considerations and Caveats* (2008)

181. E. Taboada, E. Rodríguez, A. Roig, J. Oró, A. Roch, R.N. Muller, Relaxometric and magnetic characterization of ultrasmall iron oxide nanoparticles with high magnetization. Evaluation as potential T1 magnetic resonance imaging contrast agents for molecular imaging. Langmuir **23**, 4583–4588 (2007)

182. M. Di Marco, C. Sadun, M. Port, I. Guilbert, P. Couvreur, C. Dubernet, Physicochemical characterization of ultrasmall superparamagnetic iron oxide particles (USPIO) for biomedical application as MRI contrast agents. Int. J. Nanomed. **2**, 609 (2007)

183. D. Artemov, N. Mori, B. Okollie, Z.M. Bhujwalla, MR molecular imaging of the Her-2/neu receptor in breast cancer cells using targeted iron oxide nanoparticles. Magn. Reson. Med. **49**, 403–408 (2003)

184. W. Wu, Z. Wu, T. Yu, C. Jiang, W.-S. Kim, Recent progress on magnetic iron oxide nanoparticles: synthesis, surface functional strategies and biomedical applications. Sci. Technol. Adv. Mater. **16**, 023501 (2016)

185. J.M. Perez, L. Josephson, R. Weissleder, Use of magnetic nanoparticles as nanosensors to probe for molecular interactions. ChemBioChem **5**, 261–264 (2004)

186. R. Jin, B. Lin, D. Li, H. Ai, Superparamagnetic iron oxide nanoparticles for MR imaging and therapy: design considerations and clinical applications. Curr. Opin. Pharmacol. **18**, 18–27 (2014)

187. A. Neuwelt, N. Sidhu, C.-A.A. Hu, G. Mlady, S.C. Eberhardt, L.O. Sillerud, Iron-based superparamagnetic nanoparticle contrast agents for MRI of infection and inflammation. AJR Am. J. Roentgenol. **204**, W302–W313 (2015)

188. A. Millon, S. Dickson, A. Klink, D. Izquierdo-Garcia, J. Bini, E. Lancelot, S. Ballet. P. Robert, J.M. de Castro, C. Corot, Monitoring plaque inflammation in atherosclerotic rabbits with an iron oxide (P904) and 18 F-FDG using a combined PET/MR scanner Atherosclerosis **228**, 339–345 (2013)

189. M.J. Jacobin-Valat, K. Deramchia, S. Mornet, C.E. Hagemeyer, S. Bonetto, R. Robert, M. Biran, P. Massot, S. Miraux, S. Sanchez, MRI of inducible P-selectin expression in human activated platelets involved in the early stages of atherosclerosis. NMR Biomed. **24**, 413–424 (2011)

190. M.A. Busquets, R. Sabaté, J. Estelrich, Potential applications of magnetic particles to detect and treat Alzheimer's disease. Nanoscale Res. Lett. **9**, 1–10 (2014)

191. M.M. Vellinga, R.D.O. Engberink, A. Seewann, P.J. Pouwels, M.P. Wattjes, S.M. van der Pol, C. Pering, C.H. Polman, H.E. de Vries, J.J. Geurts, Pluriformity of inflammation in multiple sclerosis shown by ultra-small iron oxide particle enhancement. Brain **131**, 800–807 (2008)

192. J. Xie, K. Chen, J. Huang, S. Lee, J. Wang, J. Gao, X. Li, X. Chen, PET/NIRF/MRI triple functional iron oxide nanoparticles. Biomaterials **31**, 3016–3022 (2010)

193. O. Veiseh, C. Sun, J. Gunn, N. Kohler, P. Gabikian, D. Lee, N. Bhattarai, R. Ellenbogen, R. Sze, A. Hallahan, Optical and MRI multifunctional nanoprobe for targeting gliomas. Nano Lett. **5**, 1003–1008 (2005)

194. H. Lee, M.K. Yu, S. Park, S. Moon, J.J. Min, Y.Y. Jeong, H.-W. Kang, S. Jon, Thermally cross-linked superparamagnetic iron oxide nanoparticles: synthesis and application as a dual imaging probe for cancer in vivo. J. Am. Chem. Soc. **129**, 12739–12745 (2007)

195. Y. Wang, X. Xie, X. Wang, G. Ku, K.L. Gill, D.P. O'Neal, G. Stoica, L.V. Wang, Photoacoustic tomography of a nanoshell contrast agent in the in vivo rat brain. Nano Lett. **4**, 1689–1692 (2004)

196. M.J. Welch, C.J. Hawker, K.L. Wooley, The advantages of nanoparticles for PET. J. Nucl. Med. **50**, 1743–1746 (2009)

197. N. Lee, S.H. Choi, T. Hyeon, Nano-Sized CT Contrast Agents. Adv. Mater. **25**, 2641–2660 (2013)

198. S. Narayanan, B.N. Sathy, U. Mony, M. Koyakutty, S.V. Nair, D. Menon, Biocompatible magnetite/gold nanohybrid contrast agents via green chemistry for MRI and CT bioimaging. ACS Appl. Mater. Interfaces **4**, 251–260 (2011)

199. J. Liu, W. Zhang, H. Zhang, Z. Yang, T. Li, B. Wang, X. Huo, R. Wang, H. Chen, A multifunctional nanoprobe based on Au–Fe$_3$O$_4$ nanoparticles for multimodal and ultrasensitive detection of cancer cells. Chem. Commun. **49**, 4938–4940 (2013)

200. Z. Liu, T. Lammers, J. Ehling, S. Fokong, J. Bornemann, F. Kiessling, J. Gätjens, Iron oxide nanoparticle-containing microbubble composites as contrast agents for MR and ultrasound dual-modality imaging. Biomaterials **32**, 6155–6163 (2011)

201. F. Kiessling, J. Huppert, M. Palmowski, Functional and molecular ultrasound imaging: concepts and contrast agents. Curr. Med. Chem. **16**, 627–642 (2009)

202. R. Misra, S. Acharya, S.K. Sahoo, Cancer nanotechnology: application of nanotechnology in cancer therapy. Drug Discov. Today **15**, 842–850 (2010)

203. U. Ikoba, H. Peng, H. Li, C. Miller, C. Yu, Q. Wang, Nanocarriers in therapy of infectious and inflammatory diseases. Nanoscale **7**, 4291–4305 (2015)

204. O. Veiseh, B.C. Tang, K.A. Whitehead, D.G. Anderson, R. Langer, Managing diabetes with nanomedicine: challenges and opportunities. Nat. Rev. Drug Discov. **14**, 45–57 (2015)

205. A.S. Gupta, Nanomedicine approaches in vascular disease: a review, Nanomedicine: Nanotechnology. Biol. Med. **7**, 763–779 (2011)

206. S. Roussakow, The history of hyperthermia rise and decline, in *Conference Papers in Science, Hindawi Publishing Corporation, 2013* (2013) p. 428027

207. O.S. Nielsen, M. Horsman, J. Overgaard, A future for hyperthermia in cancer treatment? Eur. J. Cancer **37**, 1587–1589 (2001)

208. S. Mornet, S. Vasseur, F. Grasset, P. Veverka, G. Goglio, A. Demourgues, J. Portier, E. Pollert, E. Duguet, Magnetic nanoparticle design for medical applications. Prog. Solid State Chem. **34**, 237–247 (2006)

209. P. Moroz, S. Jones, B. Gray, Magnetically mediated hyperthermia: current status and future directions. Int. J. Hyperth. **18**, 267–284 (2002)

210. A. Jordan, R. Scholz, K. Maier-Hauff, M. Johannsen, P. Wust, J. Nadobny, H. Schirra, H. Schmidt, S. Deger, S. Loening, Presentation of a new magnetic field therapy system for the treatment of human solid tumors with magnetic fluid hyperthermia. J. Magn. Magn. Mater. **225**, 118–126 (2001)
211. A.E. Deatsch, B.A. Evans, Heating efficiency in magnetic nanoparticle hyperthermia. J. Magn. Magn. Mater. **354**, 163–172 (2014)
212. C.S. Kumar, F. Mohammad, Magnetic nanomaterials for hyperthermia-based therapy and controlled drug delivery. Adv. Drug Deliv. Rev. **63**, 789–808 (2011)
213. M.F.X. Gnant, E.M. Turner, H.R. Alexander, Effects of hyperthermia and tumour necrosis factor on inflammatory cytokine secretion and procoagulant activity in endothelial cells. Cytokine **12**, 339–347 (2000)
214. B. Hildebrandt, P. Wust, O. Ahlers, A. Dieing, G. Sreenivasa, T. Kerner, R. Felix, H. Riess, The cellular and molecular basis of hyperthermia. Critical Rev. Oncol./Hematol. **43**, 33–56 (2002)
215. E. Kita, T. Oda, T. Kayano, S. Sato, M. Minagawa, H. Yanagihara, M. Kishimoto, C. Mitsumata, S. Hashimoto, K. Yamada, Ferromagnetic nanoparticles for magnetic hyperthermia and thermoablation therapy. J. Phys. D Appl. Phys. **43**, 474011 (2010)
216. T.L. Kalber, K.L. Ordidge, P. Southern, M.R. Loebinger, P.G. Kyrtatos, Q.A. Pankhurst, M.F. Lythgoe, S.M. Janes, Hyperthermia treatment of tumors by mesenchymal stem cell-delivered superparamagnetic iron oxide nanoparticles. Int. J. Nanomed. **11**, 1973–1983 (2016)
217. V.P. Torchilin, Multifunctional, stimuli-sensitive nanoparticulate systems for drug delivery. Nat. Rev. Drug Discov. **13**, 813–827 (2014)
218. M. Hans, A. Lowman, Biodegradable nanoparticles for drug delivery and targeting. Curr. Opin. Solid State Mater. Sci. **6**, 319–327 (2002)
219. O.C. Farokhzad, R. Langer, Impact of nanotechnology on drug delivery. ACS Nano **3**, 16–20 (2009)
220. S.S. Suri, H. Fenniri, B. Singh, Nanotechnology-based drug delivery systems. J. Occup. Med. Toxicol. **2**, 1–6 (2007)
221. H. Maeda, J. Wu, T. Sawa, Y. Matsumura, K. Hori, Tumor vascular permeability and the EPR effect in macromolecular therapeutics: a review. J. Controlled Release **65**, 271–284 (2000)
222. F. Danhier, O. Feron, V. Préat, To exploit the tumor microenvironment: passive and active tumor targeting of nanocarriers for anti-cancer drug delivery. J. Controlled Release **148**, 135–146 (2010)
223. F. Chen, H. Hong, Y. Zhang, H.F. Valdovinos, S. Shi, G.S. Kwon, C.P. Theuer, T.E. Barnhart, W. Cai, In vivo tumor targeting and image-guided drug delivery with antibody-conjugated, radiolabeled mesoporous silica nanoparticles. ACS Nano **7**, 9027–9039 (2013)
224. O.C. Farokhzad, J. Cheng, B.A. Teply, I. Sherifi, S. Jon, P.W. Kantoff, J.P. Richie, R. Langer, Targeted nanoparticle-aptamer bioconjugates for cancer chemotherapy in vivo. Proc. Natl. Acad. Sci. **103**, 6315–6320 (2006)
225. M. Muthiah, I.-K. Park, C.-S. Cho, Surface modification of iron oxide nanoparticles by biocompatible polymers for tissue imaging and targeting. Biotechnol. Adv. **31**, 1224–1236 (2013)
226. B. Chertok, B.A. Moffat, A.E. David, F. Yu, C. Bergemann, B.D. Ross, V.C. Yang, Iron oxide nanoparticles as a drug delivery vehicle for MRI monitored magnetic targeting of brain tumors. Biomaterials **29**, 487–496 (2008)
227. O. Veiseh, J.W. Gunn, M. Zhang, Design and fabrication of magnetic nanoparticles for targeted drug delivery and imaging. Adv. Drug Deliv. Rev. **62**, 284–304 (2010)
228. A. Zarrin, S. Sadighian, K. Rostamizadeh, O. Firuzi, M. Hamidi, S. Mohammadi-Samani, R. Miri, Design, preparation, and in vitro characterization of a trimodally-targeted nanomagnetic onco-theranostic system for cancer diagnosis and therapy. Int. J. Pharm. **500**, 62–76 (2016)

229. B. Polyak, G. Friedman, Magnetic targeting for site-specific drug delivery: applications and clinical potential. Expert Opin. Drug Deliv. **6**, 53–70 (2009)
230. C. de las Heras Alarcón, S. Pennadam, C. Alexander, Stimuli responsive polymers for biomedical applications. Chem. Soc. Rev. **34**, 276–285 (2005)
231. J. Chomoucka, J. Drbohlavova, D. Huska, V. Adam, R. Kizek, J. Hubalek, Magnetic nanoparticles and targeted drug delivering. Pharmacol. Res. **62**, 144–149 (2010)
232. M. Mikhaylova, D.K. Kim, N. Bobrysheva, M. Osmolowsky, V. Semenov, T. Tsakalakos, M. Muhammed, Superparamagnetism of magnetite nanoparticles: dependence on surface modification. Langmuir **20**, 2472–2477 (2004)
233. S.K. Yen, P. Padmanabhan, S.T. Selvan, Multifunctional iron oxide nanoparticles for diagnostics, therapy and macromolecule delivery. Theranostics **3**, 986–1003 (2013)
234. L. Zhao, T. Chano, S. Morikawa, Y. Saito, A. Shiino, S. Shimizu, T. Maeda, T. Irie, S. Aonuma, H. Okabe, Hyperbranched polyglycerol-grafted superparamagnetic iron oxide nanoparticles: synthesis, characterization, functionalization, size separation, magnetic properties, and biological applications. Adv. Funct. Mater. **22**, 5107–5117 (2012)
235. A.A. Moghanjoughi, D. Khoshnevis, A. Zarrabi, A concise review on smart polymers for controlled drug release. Drug Deliv. Transl. Res. **6**, 333–340 (2016)
236. H. Mousavi, B. Movahedi, A. Zarrabi, M. Jahandar, A multifunctional hierarchically assembled magnetic nanostructure towards cancer nano-theranostics. RSC Adv. **5**, 77255–77263 (2015)
237. N. Kamaly, A.D. Miller, Paramagnetic liposome nanoparticles for cellular and tumour imaging. Int. J. Mol. Sci. **11**, 1759–1776 (2010)
238. N.G. Durmus, E.N. Taylor, K.M. Kummer, T.J. Webster, Enhanced efficacy of superparamagnetic iron oxide nanoparticles against antibiotic-resistant biofilms in the presence of metabolites. Adv. Mater. **25**, 5706–5713 (2013)
239. J.H. Maeng, D.-H. Lee, K.H. Jung, Y.-H. Bae, I.-S. Park, S. Jeong, Y.-S. Jeon, C.-K. Shim, W. Kim, J. Kim, Multifunctional doxorubicin loaded superparamagnetic iron oxide nanoparticles for chemotherapy and magnetic resonance imaging in liver cancer. Biomaterials **31**, 4995–5006 (2010)
240. F.M. Kievit, F.Y. Wang, C. Fang, H. Mok, K. Wang, J.R. Silber, R.G. Ellenbogen, M. Zhang, Doxorubicin loaded iron oxide nanoparticles overcome multidrug resistance in cancer in vitro. J. Controlled Release **152**, 76–83 (2011)
241. O. Mykhaylyk, Y.S. Antequera, D. Vlaskou, C. Plank, Generation of magnetic nonviral gene transfer agents and magnetofection in vitro. Nat. Protoc. **2**, 2391–2411 (2007)
242. S. Govindarajan, K. Kitaura, M. Takafuji, H. Ihara, K. Varadarajan, A.B. Patel, V. Gopal, Gene delivery into human cancer cells by cationic lipid-mediated magnetofection. Int. J. Pharm. **446**, 87–99 (2013)
243. U. Schillinger, T. Brill, C. Rudolph, S. Huth, S. Gersting, F. Krötz, J. Hirschberger, C. Bergemann, C. Plank, Advances in magnetofection—magnetically guided nucleic acid delivery. J. Magn. Magn. Mater. **293**, 501–508 (2005)
244. P. Jendelová, V. Herynek, J. DeCroos, K. Glogarová, B. Andersson, M. Hájek, E. Syková, Imaging the fate of implanted bone marrow stromal cells labeled with superparamagnetic nanoparticles. Magn. Reson. Med. **50**, 767–776 (2003)
245. D.K. Kirui, D.A. Rey, C.A. Batt, Gold hybrid nanoparticles for targeted phototherapy and cancer imaging. Nanotechnology **21**, 105105 (2010)
246. M. Chu, Y. Shao, J. Peng, X. Dai, H. Li, Q. Wu, D. Shi, Near-infrared laser light mediated cancer therapy by photothermal effect of Fe_3O_4 magnetic nanoparticles. Biomaterials **34**, 4078–4088 (2013)
247. M. Thandu, V. Rapozzi, L. Xodo, F. Albericio, C. Comuzzi, S. Cavalli, "Clicking" porphyrins to magnetic nanoparticles for photodynamic therapy. ChemPlusChem **79**, 90–98 (2014)
248. D.B. Tada, L.L. Vono, E.L. Duarte, R. Itri, P.K. Kiyohara, M.S. Baptista, L.M. Rossi, Methylene blue-containing silica-coated magnetic particles: a potential magnetic carrier for photodynamic therapy. Langmuir **23**, 8194–8199 (2007)

249. A.E. Fard, A. Zarepour, A. Zarrabi, A. Shanei, H. Salehi, Synergistic effect of the combination of triethylene-glycol modified Fe_3O_4 nanoparticles and ultrasound wave on MCF-7 cells. J. Magn. Magn. Mater. **394**, 44–49 (2015)

250. H. Xu, X. Zhang, R. Han, P. Yang, H. Ma, Y. Song, Z. Lu, W. Yin, X. Wu, H. Wang, Nanoparticles in sonodynamic therapy: state of the art review. RSC Advances **6**, 50697–50705 (2016)

251. C. Tassa, S.Y. Shaw, R. Weissleder, Dextran-coated iron oxide nanoparticles: a versatile platform for targeted molecular imaging, molecular diagnostics, and therapy. Acc. Chem. Res. **44**, 842–852 (2011)

252. H.-M. Yang, B.C. Oh, J.H. Kim, T. Ahn, H.-S. Nam, C.W. Park, J.-D. Kim, Multifunctional poly (aspartic acid) nanoparticles containing iron oxide nanocrystals and doxorubicin for simultaneous cancer diagnosis and therapy. Colloids Surf., A **391**, 208–215 (2011)

253. H. Xu, L. Cheng, C. Wang, X. Ma, Y. Li, Z. Liu, Polymer encapsulated upconversion nanoparticle/iron oxide nanocomposites for multimodal imaging and magnetic targeted drug delivery. Biomaterials **32**, 9364–9373 (2011)

254. M. Jahandar, A. Zarrabi, M.A. Shokrgozar, H. Mousavi, Synthesis, characterization and application of polyglycerol coated Fe_3O_4 nanoparticles as a nano-theranostics agent. Mater. Res. Express **2**, 125002 (2015)

255. N. Nasongkla, E. Bey, J. Ren, H. Ai, C. Khemtong, J.S. Guthi, S.-F. Chin, A.D. Sherry, D.A. Boothman, J. Gao, Multifunctional polymeric micelles as cancer-targeted, MRI-ultrasensitive drug delivery systems. Nano Lett. **6**, 2427–2430 (2006)

256. H. Guo, W. Chen, X. Sun, Y.-N. Liu, J. Li, J. Wang, Theranostic magnetoliposomes coated by carboxymethyl dextran with controlled release by low-frequency alternating magnetic field. Carbohydr. Polym. **118**, 209–217 (2015)

257. Q. Quan, J. Xie, H. Gao, M. Yang, F. Zhang, G. Liu, X. Lin, A. Wang, H.S. Eden, S. Lee, HSA coated iron oxide nanoparticles as drug delivery vehicles for cancer therapy. Mol. Pharm. **8**, 1669–1676 (2011)

258. K. Cheng, S. Peng, C. Xu, S. Sun, Porous hollow Fe3O4 nanoparticles for targeted delivery and controlled release of cisplatin. J. Am. Chem. Soc. **131**, 10637–10644 (2009)

259. C. Wang, S. Ravi, U.S. Garapati, M. Das, M. Howell, J. Mallela, S. Alwarappan, S.S. Mohapatra, S. Mohapatra, Multifunctional chitosan magnetic-graphene (CMG) nanoparticles: a theranostic platform for tumor-targeted co-delivery of drugs, genes and MRI contrast agents. J. Mater. Chem. B **1**, 4396–4405 (2013)

260. H. Yang, Y. Li, T. Li, M. Xu, Y. Chen, C. Wu, X. Dang, Y. Liu, Multifunctional core/shell nanoparticles cross-linked polyetherimide-folic acid as efficient Notch-1 siRNA carrier for targeted killing of breast cancer. Sci. Rep. **4**, 7072 (2014)

261. M.K. Jaiswal, M. De, S.S. Chou, S. Vasavada, R. Bleher, P.V. Prasad, D. Bahadur, V.P. Dravid, Thermoresponsive magnetic hydrogels as theranostic nanoconstructs. ACS Appl. Mater. Interfaces **6**, 6237–6247 (2014)

262. M.M. Yallapu, S.F. Othman, E.T. Curtis, B.K. Gupta, M. Jaggi, S.C. Chauhan, Multi-functional magnetic nanoparticles for magnetic resonance imaging and cancer therapy. Biomaterials **32**, 1890–1905 (2011)

263. G.R. Reddy, M.S. Bhojani, P. McConville, J. Moody, B.A. Moffat, D.E. Hall, G. Kim, Y.-E.L. Koo, M.J. Woolliscroft, J.V. Sugai, Vascular targeted nanoparticles for imaging and treatment of brain tumors. Clin. Cancer Res. **12**, 6677–6686 (2006)

264. K. Yang, L. Hu, X. Ma, S. Ye, L. Cheng, X. Shi, C. Li, Y. Li, Z. Liu, Multimodal imaging guided photothermal therapy using functionalized graphene nanosheets anchored with magnetic nanoparticles. Adv. Mater. **24**, 1868–1872 (2012)

265. Z. Zhou, Y. Sun, J. Shen, J. Wei, C. Yu, B. Kong, W. Liu, H. Yang, S. Yang, W. Wang, Iron/iron oxide core/shell nanoparticles for magnetic targeting MRI and near-infrared photothermal therapy. Biomaterials **35**, 7470–7478 (2014)

266. L. Cheng, K. Yang, Y. Li, X. Zeng, M. Shao, S.-T. Lee, Z. Liu, Multifunctional nanoparticles for upconversion luminescence/MR multimodal imaging and magnetically targeted photothermal therapy. Biomaterials **33**, 2215–2222 (2012)

267. W. Dong, Y. Li, D. Niu, Z. Ma, J. Gu, Y. Chen, W. Zhao, X. Liu, C. Liu, J. Shi, Facile synthesis of monodisperse superparamagnetic Fe_3O_4 core@hybrid@Au shell nanocomposite for bimodal imaging and photothermal therapy. Adv. Mater. **23**, 5392–5397 (2011)

268. H.-Y. Huang, S.-H. Hu, S.-Y. Hung, C.-S. Chiang, H.-L. Liu, T.-L. Chiu, H.-Y. Lai, Y.-Y. Chen, S.-Y. Chen, SPIO nanoparticle-stabilized PAA-F127 thermosensitive nanobubbles with MR/US dual-modality imaging and HIFU-triggered drug release for magnetically guided in vivo tumor therapy. J. Controlled Release **172**, 118–127 (2013)

269. J. Huang, M. Guo, H. Ke, C. Zong, B. Ren, G. Liu, H. Shen, Y. Ma, X. Wang, H. Zhang, Rational Design and Synthesis of γFe_2O_3@Au Magnetic Gold Nanoflowers for Efficient Cancer Theranostics. Adv. Mater. **27**, 5049–5056 (2015)

270. D. Calle, V. Negri, P. Ballesteros, S. Cerdán, Magnetoliposomes loaded with poly-unsaturated fatty acids as novel theranostic anti-inflammatory formulations. Theranostics (2015)

271. T. Fu, Q. Kong, H. Sheng, L. Gao, Value of functionalized superparamagnetic iron oxide nanoparticles in the diagnosis and treatment of acute temporal lobe epilepsy on MRI. Neural Plast. **2016**, 2412958 (2016)

272. L. Moraes, A. Vasconcelos-dos-Santos, F.C. Santana, M.A. Godoy, P.H. Rosado-de-Castro, R.L. Azevedo-Pereira, W.M. Cintra, E.L. Gasparetto, M.F. Santiago, R. Mendez-Otero, Neuroprotective effects and magnetic resonance imaging of mesenchymal stem cells labeled with SPION in a rat model of Huntington's disease. Stem Cell Res. **9**, 143–155 (2012)

273. P. Wang, M.V. Yigit, Z. Medarova, L. Wei, G. Dai, C. Schuetz, A. Moore, Combined small interfering RNA therapy and in vivo magnetic resonance imaging in islet transplantation. Diabetes **60**, 565–571 (2011)

274. N. Ahmed, H. Fessi, A. Elaissari, Theranostic applications of nanoparticles in cancer. Drug Discov. Today **17**, 928–934 (2012)

275. C. von Zur, D.Von Muhlen, N. Elverfeldt, I. Bassler, B. Neudorfer, A. Steitz, H. Petri-Fink, C. Hofmann, K. Bode, Peter, Superparamagnetic iron oxide binding and uptake as imaged by magnetic resonance is mediated by the integrin receptor Mac-1 (CD11b/CD18): implications on imaging of atherosclerotic plaques. Atherosclerosis **193**, 102–111 (2007)

276. M. Lundqvist, J. Stigler, G. Elia, I. Lynch, T. Cedervall, K.A. Dawson, Nanoparticle size and surface properties determine the protein corona with possible implications for biological impacts. Proc. Natl. Acad. Sci. **105**, 14265–14270 (2008)

277. A. Lesniak, A. Salvati, M.J. Santos-Martinez, M.W. Radomski, K.A. Dawson, C. Åberg, Nanoparticle adhesion to the cell membrane and its effect on nanoparticle uptake efficiency. J. Am. Chem. Soc. **135**, 1438–1444 (2013)

278. A.K. Gupta, M. Gupta, Cytotoxicity suppression and cellular uptake enhancement of surface modified magnetic nanoparticles. Biomaterials **26**, 1565–1573 (2005)

279. L.L. Muldoon, M. Sàndor, K.E. Pinkston, E.A. Neuwelt, Imaging, distribution, and toxicity of superparamagnetic iron oxide magnetic resonance nanoparticles in the rat brain and intracerebral tumor. Neurosurgery **57**, 785–796 (2005)

280. M. Mahmoudi, A. Simchi, A. Milani, P. Stroeve, Cell toxicity of superparamagnetic iron oxide nanoparticles. J. Colloid Interface Sci. **336**, 510–518 (2009)

281. F. Dilnawaz, S.K. Sahoo, Therapeutic approaches of magnetic nanoparticles for the central nervous system. Drug Discovery Today **20**, 1256–1264 (2015)

282. G. Huang, H. Chen, Y. Dong, X. Luo, H. Yu, Z. Moore, E.A. Bey, D.A. Boothman, J. Gao, Superparamagnetic iron oxide nanoparticles: amplifying ROS stress to improve anticancer drug efficacy. Theranostics **3**, 116–126 (2013)

283. L. Zeng, Z. Shen, A. Wu, Magnetic nanomaterials for tumor targeting theranostics. Nanomater. Tumor Targ. Theranostics: A Proact. Clin. Perspect. (2016) 55